RAPID

PEDIATRIC

Emergency Care

Revised Edition

Barbara Aehlert, RN, BSPA

Southwest EMS Education, Inc.
Phoenix, Arizona/Pursley, Texas

ELSEVIER

MOSBY JEMS
ELSEVIER

11830 Westline Industrial Drive
St. Louis, Missouri 63146

RAPID Pediatric Emergency   ISBN-13   978-0-323-04747-0
Care, Revised Edition   ISBN   0-323-04747-5
Copyright © 2007, Mosby, Inc. All rights reserved.

NOTICE

Knowledge and best practice in this field are constantly changing. As
new research and experience broaden our knowledge, changes in
practice, treatment, and drug therapy may become necessary or
appropriate. Readers are advised to check the most current information
provided (i) on procedures featured or (ii) by the manufacturer of each
product to be administered, to verify the recommended dose or
formula, the method and duration of administration, and
contraindications. It is the responsibility of the practitioners, relying on
their own experience and knowledge of the patient, to make diagnoses,
to determine dosages, to identify the best treatment for each individual
patient, and to take all appropriate safety precautions. To the fullest
extent of the law, neither the Publisher nor the Author or Editors
assume any liability for any injury and/or damage to persons or
property arising out of or related to any use of the material contained
in this book

Executive Editor: Linda Honeycutt
Developmental Editor: Katherine Tomber
Publishing Services Manager: Julie Eddy
Senior Project Manager: JoAnn Amore
Cover Design: Paula Ruckenbrod

Printed in China

Last digit is the print number: 9 8 7 6 5 4 3 2 1

■ A&P and CARE CONSIDERATIONS ■

BIRTH TO 1 MONTH

- Anatomic and physiologic considerations
  - ▸ At birth, the neonate's head accounts for 1/4 of the body length and 1/3 of the body weight. Because of the neonate's large occiput, it is easy to hyperextend or flex the neck, compromising the airway.
  - ▸ At birth, the ribs are composed mainly of cartilage and project at right angles from the vertebral column. As a result, the ribcage is more circular than in adults.
  - ▸ Muscle mass makes up about 25% of birth weight.
  - ▸ Cranial bones are soft and separated by sutures. Membranous spaces (fontanelles) between the cranial bones allow expansion of the skull to accommodate brain growth. Vaginal delivery often causes molding of the neonate's skull, during which the cranial bones may shift and overlap. The skull resumes its appropriate size and shape within days.
  - ▸ The neonate's body, particularly the shoulders and back, may be covered with lanugo (fine, silky hair). Most of this hair is shed within 10 to 14 days.
  - ▸ Neonates are obligatory nose breathers. Complete or partial obstruction often results in respiratory distress.

- ▶ Neonates are predisposed to hypothermia because of their small mass, large ratio of surface area to weight, and poor development of the subcutaneous fat layer of the skin.
- ▶ Limited glycogen stores predispose the neonate to hypoglycemia.
- Emergency care implications
  - ▶ Observe the baby before making contact.
  - ▶ Keep in caregiver's arms if possible.
  - ▶ Handle patient gently, but firmly, supporting the head and neck.
    - ○ **Do not shake or jiggle the baby**.
    - ○ A one-per-second swaying motion is comforting.
  - ▶ Perform least invasive parts of the examination first.
  - ▶ Keep the baby warm; warm anything that touches the baby, such as hands, stethoscope, or blankets; keep the baby covered when not being examined.
  - ▶ Speak softly and smile.
  - ▶ Allow pacifier for comfort.
  - ▶ Avoid loud noises, bright lights, and abrupt, jerky movements.

INFANT (1 TO 12 MONTHS)

- Anatomic and physiologic considerations
  - ▶ The birth weight of most infants doubles within 5 months and triples within a year.
  - ▶ The three fetal shunts (ductus venosus, foramen ovale, and ductus arteriosus) normally close at birth or soon after.
  - ▶ Infants under 6 months are obligate nose breathers. Any degree of obstruction (e.g., swelling of the nasal mucosa, accumulation of mucus) can result in

respiratory difficulty and problems with feeding.

- ► A small degree of airway edema can be significant because of the small diameter of the airway, resulting in disproportionately higher resistance to airflow than in an adult.
- ► An infant's vocal cords are more cartilaginous than an adult's and are easily damaged.
- ► An infant's chest wall is thin, and the bony and cartilaginous rib cage is soft and pliant. Breathing is predominantly a result of diaphragmatic movement. Impaired movement of the diaphragm, such as that resulting from gastric distention, can significantly affect ventilation. Because of an infant's thin chest wall, transmitted breath sounds make localizing a problem area difficult.
- ► Infants in the first 3 months of life have an immature immunologic system and are more susceptible to severe infections and to infections by unusual organisms than is an older infant or child.
- ► Salivation starts at about 3 months Drooling continues until the infant's swallowing reflex is more coordinated.
- ► The midpoint in the height of an infant is the umbilicus, whereas the midpoint of an adult occurs at the symphysis pubis.
- ► Infants have a higher circulating blood volume (about 75 mL/kg) compared to that of an adult (55 to 75 mL/kg).
- ► The anterior and posterior fontanelles are membranous spaces formed where four cranial bones meet and intersect. Pulsations of the fontanelle reflect the heart rate. The posterior fontanelle usually closes by 2 months of age.

In most infants, the anterior fontanelle closes between 7 and 14 months of age. A bulging anterior fontanelle may result from crying, coughing, vomiting, or increased intracranial pressure (ICP) due to a head injury, meningitis, or hydrocephalus. A depressed anterior fontanelle is seen in dehydrated or malnourished infants.

- Subcutaneous fat reaches a maximum thickness in children 9 months of age. This is reflected in the difficulty of placing a peripheral IV line at this age.
- An infant's abdomen is protuberant because of poorly developed abdominal muscles. The liver is proportionately larger in the abdominal cavity than is the liver of an adult.
- Underdeveloped cervical ligaments, relatively weak neck muscles, and anteriorly wedged cervical vertebrae make an infant susceptible to extreme hyperflexion and hyperextension of the neck and greater head motion when subjected to acceleration-deceleration forces.

• Common fears
  - Separation from primary caregiver
  - Stranger anxiety (crying or being wary of strangers)

• Emergency care implications
  - Observe the infant before making contact.
  - Keep the infant on the caregiver's lap during physical examination if possible.
  - Handle the patient gently but firmly, supporting the head and neck.
    ○ **Do not shake or jiggle the infant.**
  - Keep the caregiver in sight if possible to decrease separation anxiety, and involve

the caregiver in care of the infant whenever possible.

▶ Return the infant to the caregiver as soon as possible after procedures; allow the caregiver to comfort.

▶ Perform least invasive parts of the examination first.

▶ Keep the infant and the environment warm; warm anything that touches the infant (e.g., hands, stethoscope).

▶ Speak softly and smile; touch, rock, hold, or cuddle if possible.

▶ Examine from toes to head.

▶ Provide comfort measures (e.g., pacifier).

▶ Distract with keys, penlight, or musical toy in the infant's field of vision.

▶ Persistent crying, irritability, or inability to console or arouse the patient may indicate physiologic distress.

TODDLER (1 TO 3 YEARS)

- Anatomic and physiologic considerations

  ▶ Trachea is small and short; may result in intubation of the right mainstem bronchus or inadvertent extubation.

  ▶ Thin chest wall allows for easily transmitted breath sounds; easy to miss a pneumothorax or misplaced tracheal tube because of transmitted breath sounds.

  ▶ Increased risk of head injuries from falls and motor vehicle crashes because of higher center of gravity.

  ▶ Children younger than 3 years are much less likely to have serious injuries than older children who fall the same distance. It is thought that younger children may better dissipate the energy transferred by the fall because they have more fat and cartilage and less muscle mass than older children.

- ► Toddlers have a higher incidence of multiple organ injury from trauma than adults because kinetic injury is dissipated into a smaller mass.
- ► On auscultation, breath sounds are louder and harsher than in an adult because of the child's relative lack of musculature and subcutaneous tissue over the thorax.
- ► The young child is particularly prone to temperature extremes because thermoregulatory controls are not completely developed.
- ► Body surface area is larger than in an adult, predisposing the child to increased heat loss through radiation, convection, and conduction.
- Common fears
  - ► Being left alone
  - ► Interacting with strangers
  - ► Interruptions in usual routine
  - ► Losing control
  - ► Getting hurt (e.g., falls, cuts, abrasions)
- Emergency care implications—examine as for infant plus:
  - ► Encourage the child's trust by gaining cooperation of caregiver.
  - ► Try not to separate the child from the caregiver.
  - ► Address the child by name.
  - ► Smile and speak in calm, quiet tone.
  - ► Allow the child to participate in care when possible.
  - ► Respect modesty; keep the child covered if possible and replace clothing promptly after examining each body area.
  - ► Allow the child to hold a transitional

object such as a blanket, doll, stuffed animal, or toy to help him or her feel secure.
- ▸ Explain that illness or injury is not the child's fault.
- ▸ Reassure the child if a procedure will not hurt.
- ▸ Do not show needles or scissors unless necessary.
- ▸ Avoid procedures on the dominant hand or arm.
- ▸ Avoid covering the child's face.
- ▸ Involve the caregiver in the treatment whenever possible.
- ▸ Persistent irritability and inability to console or arouse patient may indicate physiologic distress.
- ▸ Foreign body airway obstruction continues to be a risk

PRESCHOOLER (3 TO 5 YEARS)

- Anatomic and physiologic considerations
  - ▸ Ribs and sternum are pliable and more resistant to rib fractures than in adults, although the force of the injury is readily transmitted to the delicate tissues of the lung and may result in a pulmonary contusion, hemothorax, or pneumothorax.
  - ▸ Preschooler cannot sustain rapid respiratory rates for long periods due to immature intercostal muscles.
  - ▸ Oxygen requirements are approximately twice those of adolescents and adults (6 to 8 mL/kg/min in a child; 3 to 4 mL/kg/min in an adult).
  - ▸ Children have a proportionately smaller functional residual capacity, and therefore proportionately smaller oxygen reserves. Hypoxia develops rapidly

because of increased oxygen requirements and decreased oxygen reserves.

- ▶ The liver and spleen of a small child are lower in the abdomen and less protected by the rib cage.
- ▶ A young child's vertebral column may withstand traction and torsion without evidence of deformity, while the spinal cord tears.
- Common fears
  - ▶ Bodily injury and mutilation
  - ▶ Loss of control
  - ▶ The unknown and the dark
  - ▶ Being left alone
  - ▶ Being lost or abandoned
  - ▶ Adults that look or act mean
- Emergency care implications—examine as for toddler plus:
  - ▶ When possible, examine and treat the child in an upright position.
  - ▶ Explain procedures in brief, simple terms as they are performed.
  - ▶ Speak quietly in clear and simple language; avoid baby talk and frightening or misleading comments (e.g., shot, deaden, cut, germs, put to sleep).
  - ▶ Allow the child to hold a transitional object or keep it in sight.
  - ▶ Tell the child what will happen next and encourage the child to help with his or her care.
  - ▶ Warn the child of a painful procedure just before carrying it out.
  - ▶ Offer the child treatment choices if possible.
  - ▶ Use an adhesive bandage after a procedure or when an injection has been given because the child may fear that

"all of my blood will leak out" if a bandage is removed or not applied.

► Respect the child's modesty.
► Keep the child warm.
► Allow the caregiver to remain with the child whenever possible to help relieve the child's fear of separation from his or her caregiver.
► Persistent irritability or inability to arouse patient may indicate physiologic distress.
► Foreign body airway obstruction risk continues.

SCHOOL-AGED CHILD (6 TO 12 YEARS)

• Anatomic and physiologic considerations
  ► Bones begin to lose flexibility around the age of 6 years, when the bony cortex begins to harden and thicken.
  ► Lung volume increases to 200 mL by age 8.
  ► In children less than 13 years old, penetrating injuries are likely to be caused by accidental impalement on objects such as scissors or picket fences, or by accidental discharge of a weapon.

• Common fears
  ► Fear of unknown setting
  ► Separation from caregiver
  ► Loss of control
  ► Pain, loss of function
  ► Bodily injury and mutilation
  ► Failure to live up to others' expectations
  ► Rejection by peers
  ► Death
  ► Being unable to compete in school, sports, or play
  ► Interruptions in daily routine

- Emergency care implications—examine as for preschooler plus:
  - Enlist the child's cooperation.
  - Introduce yourself to the child. Approach in a friendly, sympathetic manner.
  - Explain procedures before carrying them out.
  - Allow the child to see and touch samples of equipment that may be used in his or her care (e.g., medicine cup, cotton swab, tongue depressor).
  - Tell the child what will happen next and encourage the child to help with care.
  - Warn the child of a painful procedure just before carrying it out.
  - Offer the child alternatives (e.g., "It is OK to yell, but don't move").
  - Make a contract with the child ("I promise to tell you everything I am going to do if you will help me by cooperating.").
  - When speaking with the caregiver, include the child.
  - Include the child in discharge instructions.
  - Persistent irritability or inability to arouse patient may indicate physiologic distress.
  - Respect the patient's modesty.
  - Reassure the patient of body integrity.
  - Address preoccupations about death when appropriate.

ADOLESCENT (13 TO 18 YEARS)

- Anatomic and physiologic considerations
  - Children grow at a faster rate during adolescence than during any other period except infancy.
  - Sebaceous glands increase sebum production in response to increased hor-

mone levels. This gives the skin an oily appearance and predisposes the adolescent to acne.
- ► By age 10, the size and flexibility of the airway matches that of adults.
- ► Bone growth ends at age 20, when the epiphyses close.
- ► By 15 years of age, cardiac output is equal to that of an adult.
- ► Circulatory response to shock is similar to that of an adult.
- ► Breast tissue in females develops between 9 and 13 years of age. Mature adult breast tissue is achieved between 13 and 16 years of age.
- Common fears
  - ► Being left out or socially isolated
  - ► Fear of inheriting parent's problems (e.g., alcoholism, mental illness)
  - ► Early and violent death
  - ► Loss of control
  - ► Altered body image
  - ► Separation from peer group
- Emergency care implications   examine as for school-aged children, plus:
  - ► Speak in a respectful, friendly manner, as if speaking to an adult.
  - ► Obtain a history from the patient if possible.
  - ► Respect independence; address the adolescent directly.
  - ► Allow the caregiver to be involved in examination if the patient wishes.
  - ► Explain things clearly and honestly; allow time for questions.
  - ► Involve the patient in treatment whenever possible.
  - ► Respect the patient's modesty.

- Address patient concerns of body integrity or disfigurement.
- Deal with the patient tactfully and fairly.
- Provide discharge instructions to the patient.
- Vital signs approach adult values.
- Consider the possibility of substance abuse or endangerment of self or others.

Non-threatening Language

Words or phrases to avoid	Suggested substitutions
Shot, bee sting, stick	Medicine under the skin
Organ	Special place in the body
Test	See how (specify body part) is working
Incision	Special opening
Edema	Puffiness
Stretcher, gurney	Rolling bed
Stool	Child's usual term
Dye	Special medicine
Pain	Hurt, discomfort, "owie," "boo-boo"
Deaden	Numb, make sleepy
Cut, fix	Make better
Take (as in "take your temperature" and "take your blood pressure")	See how warm you are; check your pressure; hug your arm
Put to sleep, anesthesia	Special sleep
Catheter	Tube
Monitor	TV screen
Electrodes	Sticklers, ticklers
Specimen	Sample

*From Wong DL, Hockenberry-Eaton M: *Wong's essentials of pediatric nursing*, ed 6, St. Louis, 2001, Mosby.

12

INITIAL EVALUATION

SCENE SURVEY

- Hazards
  - ▶ Note any hazards or potential hazards and any visible mechanism of injury or illness.
  - ▶ Presence of pills, medicine bottles, or household chemicals may indicate a possible toxic ingestion.
  - ▶ Injury and history that does not coincide with the mechanism of injury may indicate child abuse.

- Relationships/interaction
  - ▶ Observe the interaction between the caregiver and the child and determine the appropriateness of their interaction. Does the interaction demonstrate concern, or is it angry or indifferent?
  - ▶ Other important assessments that can be made during the scene survey include:
    - ○ Orderliness, cleanliness, and safety of the home

- ○ General appearance of other children in the family
- ○ Presence of any medical devices used for the child (e.g., ventilator)
- ○ Indications of parental substance abuse
- Determine if additional resources are necessary, including law enforcement, fire equipment, extrication equipment, special rescue services, additional medical personnel, or special transport services (aeromedical transport).

PEDIATRIC ASSESSMENT COMPONENTS

In practice, some steps can be performed simultaneously, particularly if additional healthcare professionals are available to assist.

- Initial assessment
  - ► Pediatric Assessment Triangle (first impression)
  - ► Primary survey (ABCDE assessment)
  - ► Secondary survey
    - ○ Vital signs
    - ○ Focused history
    - ○ Detailed physical examination
- Ongoing assessment

INITIAL ASSESSMENT

Pediatric Assessment Triangle (PAT)

- First impression/"across-the-room" assessment
  - ► Because approaching an ill or injured child can increase agitation, possibly worsening the child's condition, the PAT is performed **before** approaching or touching the child.
  - ► Pause a short distance from the patient and, using your senses of sight and

hearing (look and listen), quickly determine if a life-threatening problem exists that requires immediate intervention

- ► Can be completed in 60 seconds or less
- ► No equipment (cardiac monitor, blood pressure cuff, stethoscope) required

PEDIATRIC ASSESSMENT TRIANGLE[19]

Appearance
Mental status
Muscle tone

Breathing
Body position
Visible movement of chest/abdomen
Work of breathing (respiratory rate/effort)
Audible airway sounds

Circulation
Skin color

- The Pediatric Assessment Triangle (PAT) and primary survey are used to quickly determine if a child is sick or not sick. Remember that your patient's condition can change at any time. A patient that initially appears not sick may deteriorate rapidly and appear sick. Reassess frequently.
  - ► Establishes severity of illness or injury (sick [unstable] or not sick [stable])
  - ► Identifies general category of physiologic abnormality (e.g., cardiopulmonary, neurologic, metabolic, toxicologic, trauma)
  - ► Determines urgency of further assessment and intervention

Appearance

- Reflects the adequacy of oxygenation, ventilation, brain perfusion, homeostasis, and central nervous system function
- Assessment areas
- Normal findings

- ▶ Normal muscle tone
- ▶ Child responds to name (if more than 6 to 8 months of age)
- ▶ Equal movement of all extremities
- ▶ Eyes open
- ▶ Normal speech or cry
- Abnormal findings

If the child exhibits abnormal findings, proceed immediately to the primary survey.

- ▶ Agitation
- ▶ Marked irritability
- ▶ Paradoxical irritability (irritable when held and lethargic when left alone; may be seen in infants and small children with neurologic infections)
- ▶ Reduced responsiveness
- ▶ Drooling (beyond infancy)
- ▶ Limp or rigid muscle tone
- ▶ Inconsolable crying
- ▶ Failure to recognize caregiver

The TICLS Assessment Tool

Tone—Is the child moving vigorously, or is the child limp, listless, or flaccid?

Interactivity—Is the child alert and attentive to his or her surroundings, or uninterested or apathetic?

Consolability—Can the child be comforted by the caregiver or healthcare professional?

Look/Gaze—Do the child's eyes follow your movement, or is there a vacant stare?

Speech/Cry—Is the child's speech or cry strong, or is it weak or hoarse?

Adapted from the American Academy of Pediatrics: Textbook of pediatric education for prehospital professionals, Sudbury, MA, 2000, Jones & Bartlett.

Breathing

- Reflects the adequacy of airway, oxygenation, and ventilation
- Assessment areas
  - ▶ Body position
  - ▶ Visible movement (chest/abdomen)
  - ▶ Respiratory rate
  - ▶ Respiratory effort
  - ▶ Audible airway sounds
- Normal findings
  - ▶ Quiet, unlabored respirations
  - ▶ Equal chest rise and fall
  - ▶ Respiratory rate within normal range
- Abnormal findings

If the child exhibits abnormal findings, proceed immediately to the primary survey

  - ▶ Abnormal body position (e.g., sniffing position, tripod position, head bobbing)
  - ▶ Nasal flaring
  - ▶ Retractions
  - ▶ Muffled or hoarse speech
  - ▶ Stridor, grunting, gasping, gurgling, or wheezing
  - ▶ Respiratory rate outside normal range
  - ▶ Accessory muscle use

Abnormal Airway Sounds

Gasping	Inhaling and exhaling with quick, difficult breaths
Grunting	Short, low-pitched sound heard at the end of exhalation that represents an attempt to generate positive end-expiratory pressure (PEEP) by exhaling against a closed glottis, prolonging the period of oxygen and carbon dioxide exchange across the alveolar-capillary membrane; a compensatory mechanism to help maintain patency of small airways and prevent atelectasis
Gurgling	Abnormal respiratory sound associated with collection of liquid or semisolid material in the patient's upper airway
Snoring	Noisy breathing through the mouth and nose during sleep, caused by air passing through a narrowed upper airway
Stridor	Harsh, high-pitched sound heard on inspiration; associated with upper airway obstruction; frequently described as a high-pitched crowing or "seal-bark" sound
Wheezing	High-pitched whistling sounds produced by air moving through narrowed airway passages

Circulation

- Reflects the adequacy of cardiac output and perfusion of vital organs (core perfusion)
- Assessment areas: skin color
- Normal findings
  - ▶ Color appears normal for child's ethnic group
- Abnormal findings

If the child exhibits abnormal findings, proceed immediately to the primary survey
  - ▶ Pallor, mottling, cyanosis

Based on your first impression, decide if the child is sick (unstable) or not sick (stable).

- If the child's condition is urgent:
  - ▶ Proceed immediately with rapid assessment of airway, breathing, and circulation
  - ▶ If a problem is identified, perform necessary interventions ("Treat as you find")
- If the child's condition is not urgent, proceed systematically:
  - ▶ Primary survey
  - ▶ Secondary survey
    - ○ Vital signs
    - ○ Focused history
    - ○ Physical examination
  - ▶ Ongoing assessment

Primary Survey

- Also called the ABCDE assessment. During the primary survey, assessment and management occur simultaneously. The primary survey should be repeated periodically, particularly after any major intervention or when a change in the patient's condition is detected.

- The primary survey focuses on basic life support (BLS) patient assessment and management. It usually requires less than 60 seconds to complete but may take longer if intervention is needed.
  - ▶ Systematic hands on assessment
  - ▶ Purpose: determine if life-threatening conditions exist
  - ▶ Components: ABCDE
    - ○ Airway and cervical spine protection
    - ○ Breathing and ventilation
    - ○ Circulation with bleeding control
    - ○ Disability (mental status)
    - ○ Exposure/environment

Airway and Cervical Spine Protection

The responsive child may have assumed a position to maximize his or her ability to maintain an open airway. Allow the child to maintain this position as you continue your assessment.

- Assessment
  - ► Goals:
    - ○ Patent airway/absence of signs or symptoms of airway obstruction (e.g., stridor, dyspnea, hoarse voice)
    - ○ Ability to handle oral secretions independently
    - ○ Patient speaks or makes appropriate sounds for age
  - ► Determine whether the airway is patent, maintainable, or unmaintainable
    - ○ Patent—able to be maintained independently
    - ○ Maintainable with positioning, suctioning
    - ○ Unmaintainable—requires assistance (e.g., tracheal intubation, cricothyrotomy, foreign body removal)
  - ► If cervical spine injury is suspected (by exam, history, or mechanism of injury), manually stabilize the head and neck in a neutral, in-line position or maintain spinal stabilization if already completed.

The head-tilt chin-lift should not be used to open the airway if trauma is suspected.

- Interventions
  - ► Spinal stabilization as needed for trauma
  - ► Jaw thrust without head tilt
  - ► Head-tilt chin-lift
  - ► Suction

- ► Reposition
- ► Removal of foreign body
- ► Airway adjuncts (e.g., oropharyngeal airway, nasopharyngeal airway)

Breathing and Ventilation

- Assessment
  - ► Goals:
    - ○ Adequate gas exchange with no signs of hypoxia
      - Awake and alert
      - Pulse oximetry = O_2 saturation >95%
      - Skin color normal; warm and dry
      - Respirations spontaneous, unlabored, and at a normal rate for age
      - Chest expansion equal bilaterally
      - Breath sounds present and clear and equal bilaterally
    - ○ Absence of dyspnea, stridor, and signs of increased work of breathing (e.g., retractions, grunting, tracheal tugging, accessory muscle use, nasal flaring, head bobbing)

Evaluation of breathing should take no more than 10 seconds.

- Confirm that the child *is* breathing and note significant abnormalities in the work of breathing. If the patient is breathing, determine if breathing is adequate or inadequate. If breathing is adequate, move on to assessment of circulation.
- Interventions
  - ► Suction
  - ► Oxygen
  - ► Airway adjuncts
  - ► Positive-pressure ventilation

Normal Respiratory Rates

AGE	BREATHS PER MINUTE (at rest)
Infant (1-12 months)	30-60
Toddler (1-3 years)	24-40
Preschooler (4-5 years)	22-34
School-age (6-12 years)	18-30
Adolescent (13-18 years)	12-16

Signs of Respiratory Distress and Respiratory Failure

RESPIRATORY DISTRESS	RESPIRATORY FAILURE
• Nasal flaring • Inspiratory retractions • Increased breathing rate (tachypnea) • Increased depth of breathing (hyperpnea) • Head-bobbing • See-saw respirations (abdominal breathing) • Restlessness • Tachycardia • Grunting • Stridor	• Cyanosis • Diminished breath sounds • Decreased level of responsiveness or response to pain • Poor skeletal muscle tone • Inadequate respiratory rate, effort, or chest excursion • Tachycardia • Use of accessory muscles of respiration

Circulation with Bleeding Control

Assessment

- Goals
  - ▶ Adequate cardiovascular function and tissue perfusion
    - ○ Awake and alert
    - ○ Central and peripheral pulses strong and regular
    - ○ Heart rate and blood pressure within normal range for age
    - ○ Skin color normal; warm and dry
    - ○ Capillary refill time is <2 seconds (assess in children <6 years of age)

- Oral intake and hydration adequate
- Urine output adequate for age and weight
  - ► Effective circulating fluid volume
    - No evidence of external bleeding
    - Vital signs within normal limits for age
    - Moist mucous membranes
    - Urine output 1 to 2 mL/kg/hour
    - Hemoglobin and hematocrit values within normal range
    - Skin turgor normal
  - ► Normal core body temperature
- Control bleeding
  - ► Look for visible external hemorrhage Control major bleeding, if present
    - Apply direct pressure over the bleeding site
    - Elevate the extremity (unless contraindicated)
    - Apply pressure over arterial pressure points
    - Apply a pressure bandage
  - ► Consider possible areas of major internal hemorrhage
    - Significant internal hemorrhage may occur in the chest, abdomen, pelvis, retroperitoneum, and femoral areas
    - Pain or swelling in any of these areas may signal possible internal hemorrhage
- Compare the strength and quality of central and peripheral pulses
  - ► Pulses can be palpated to estimate heart rate, blood pressure, cardiac output, and systemic vascular resistance

Hypotension often occurs well before the loss of central pulses.

- ► Pulse quality reflects the adequacy of peripheral perfusion.
  - ○ A weak central pulse may indicate decompensated shock.
  - ○ A peripheral pulse that is difficult to find, weak, or irregular suggests poor peripheral perfusion and may be a sign of shock or hemorrhage.
- ► Determine if the heart rate is within normal limits for the child's age. Normal heart rates by age are listed in the table on the next page.
- • Evaluate skin color, temperature, moisture
  - ► Skin turgor
    - ○ To assess skin turgor (elasticity), grasp the skin on the abdomen between your thumb and index finger. Pull the skin taut and then release quickly. Observe the speed with which the skin returns to its original contour when released.
    - ○ The skin should resume its shape immediately with no tenting or wrinkling. Good skin turgor indicates adequate hydration.
    - ○ Decreased skin turgor (a sign of dehydration and/or malnutrition) is present when the skin is released and it remains pinched (tented) and then slowly returns to its normal shape.
    - ○ Evaluate capillary refill

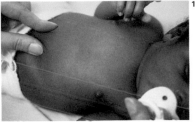

Assessing skin turgor in an infant.

Interventions

- Oxygen
- Position
- Chest compressions
- Bleeding control
- Fluid replacement
- Defibrillation

Grading of Pulses

DESCRIPTION	GRADE
Full, bounding, not obliterated with pressure	4
Normal – easily palpated, not easily obliterated with pressure	3
Difficult to palpate, obliterated with pressure	2
Weak, thready, difficult to palpate	1
Absent pulse	0

Normal Heart Rates

AGE	BEATS PER MINUTE[a]
Infant (1-12 months)	100-160
Toddler (1-3 years)	90-150
Preschooler (4-5 years)	80-140
School-age (6-12 years)	70-120
Adolescent (13-18 years)	60-100

*Pulse rates for a sleeping child may be 10% lower than the low rate listed in age group.

Disability (mental status)

Assessment

- Goal—Awake and alert
- Determine level of responsiveness, using AVPU:
  - ► A = **A**lert
  - ► V = Responds to **v**erbal stimuli
  - ► P = Responds to **p**ainful stimuli
  - ► U = **U**nresponsive
- Another assessment tool that may be used is a version of the Glasgow Coma Scale (GCS), modified for pediatric use. The pediatric GCS can be used to establish a baseline and for comparison in later, serial observations.
  - ► A GCS score that falls two points suggests significant deterioration; urgent patient reassessment is required.
  - ► To avoid confusion with spinal reflexes, assess the patient's motor response by applying a stimulus above the neck.
- Question the parent/caregiver about the child's normal mood, activity level, attention span, and willingness and ability to cooperate.

Interventions

- Oxygen
- Ventilation
- Position
- Spinal stabilization

Glasgow Coma Scale

GLASGOW COMA SCALE	ADULT/CHILD	SCORE	INFANT
Eye Opening	Spontaneous	4	Spontaneous
	To verbal	3	To verbal
	To pain	2	To pain
	No response	1	No response
Best Verbal Response	Oriented	5	Coos, babbles
	Disoriented	4	Irritable cry
	Inappropriate words	3	Cries only to pain
	Incomprehensible sounds	2	Moans to pain
	No response	1	No response
Best Motor Response	Obeys commands	6	Spontaneous
	Localizes pain	5	Withdraws from touch
	Withdraws from pain	4	Withdraws from pain
	Abnormal flexion (decorticate)	3	Abnormal flexion (decorticate)
	Abnormal extension (decerebrate)	2	Abnormal extension (decerebrate)
	No response	1	No response
	Total = **E** + **V** + **M**	3-15	

INITIAL ASSESSMENT—FIRST IMPRESSION

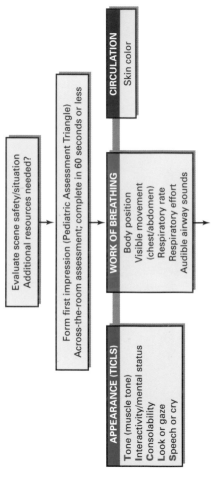

Evaluate scene safety/situation
Additional resources needed?

Form first impression (Pediatric Assessment Triangle)
Across-the-room assessment; complete in 60 seconds or less

APPEARANCE (TICLS)

Tone (muscle tone)
Interactivity/mental status
Consolability
Look or gaze
Speech or cry

WORK OF BREATHING

Body position
Visible movement
(chest/abdomen)
Respiratory rate
Respiratory effort
Audible airway sounds

CIRCULATION

Skin color

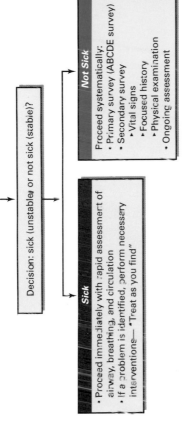

Decision: sick (unstable) or not sick (stable)?

Sick

- Proceed immediately with rapid assessment of airway, breathing, and circulation
- If a problem is identified, perform necessary interventions—"Treat as you find"

Not Sick

Proceed systematically:
- Primary survey (ABCDE survey)
- Secondary survey
  - Vital signs
  - Focused history
  - Physical examination
- Ongoing assessment

29

INITIAL ASSESSMENT—PRIMARY SURVEY (ABCDE)

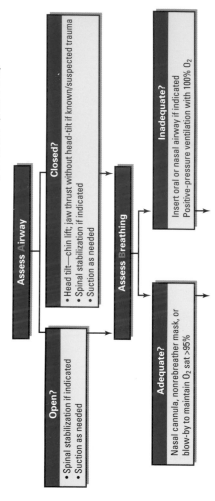

Assess Airway

Open?
- Spinal stabilization if indicated
- Suction as needed

Closed?
- Head tilt—chin lift; jaw thrust without head-tilt if known/suspected trauma
- Spinal stabilization if indicated
- Suction as needed

Assess Breathing

Adequate?
Nasal cannula, nonrebreather mask, or blow-by to maintain O₂ sat >95%

Inadequate?
Insert oral or nasal airway if indicated
Positive-pressure ventilation with 100% O₂

Assess Circulation

Pulse or other signs of circulation absent?
- Begin CPR
- Evaluate cardiac rhythm on arrival of AED/monitor/defibrillator

Electrical activity present?

Yes
- If ventricular fibrillation (VF) or ventricular tachycardia (VT): continue CPR and go to VF/VT
- If pulseless electrical activity (PEA): continue CPR and go to PEA

No
- Asystole: continue CPR and go to asystole

Pulse present?
- Control major bleeding (if present)
- Assess skin
- Assess capillary refill

Assess Disability (mental status)
- AVPU
- Pediatric Glasgow Coma Scale

Exposure/environment
- Preserve body heat
- Maintain appropriate temperature

Proceed to Secondary Survey

INITIAL ASSESSMENT—SECONDARY SURVEY

Obtain vital signs, attach pulse oximeter and blood pressure monitor

→ Obtain focused SAMPLE or CIAMPEDS history

AIRWAY
- Reassess effectiveness of initial airway maneuvers and interventions
- Perform invasive airway management if needed

BREATHING
- Reassess ventilation
- If applicable, confirm tracheal tube placement (or other airway device) by at least two methods
- Provide positive-pressure ventilation (if applicable) and evaluate effectiveness of ventilations

CIRCULATION
- Establish vascular access and administer medications, if appropriate

DETAILED (OR FOCUSED) EXAMINATION, DIFFERENTIAL DIAGNOSIS, DIAGNOSTIC PROCEDURES

- If unresponsive or there is significant mechanism of injury, perform detailed (head-to-toes) physical-exam. If responsive or there is no significant mechanism of injury, perform focused exam
  - Search for, find, and treat reversible causes
  - Glucose check
  - Laboratory and radiographic studies

EVALUATE interventions, pain management

FACILITATE family presence for invasive and resuscitative procedures

→

Perform an ongoing assessment (monitor and reassess)

- Reassess airway patency, oxygen saturation
- Reassess breathing effectiveness
- Reassess pulse rate and quality, perfusion status, cardiac rhythm
- Reassess capillary refill (if < 6 years of age)
- Reassess mental status and activity level
- Reassess and document vital signs
- Reevaluate emergency care interventions

Exposure/Environment

- Undress the patient.
- Preserve body heat and maintain appropriate temperature.
  - ▶ Respect modesty.
  - ▶ Keep the child covered if possible and replace clothing promptly after examining each body area.

Secondary Survey

The secondary survey focuses on advanced life support (ALS) interventions and management.

- Obtain vital signs, attach pulse oximeter, ECG, and blood pressure monitor
- Obtain focused SAMPLE or CIAMPEDS history
- (Advanced) *Airway*
- *Breathing*
- *Circulation*
- *Detailed* (or focused) examination, differential diagnosis, diagnostic procedures
- *Evaluate* interventions, pain management
- *Facilitate* family presence for invasive and resuscitative procedures

Lower Limit of Normal Systolic Blood Pressure	
AGE	LOWER LIMIT OF NORMAL SYSTOLIC BLOOD PRESSURE
Term neonate (0 to 28 days)	>60 mm Hg or strong central pulse
Infant (1 to 12 months)	>70 mm Hg or strong central pulse
Child 1 to 10 years	>70 + (2 x age in years)
Child ≥ 10 years	>90 mm Hg

Focused History

SAMPLE is a mnemonic used to organize the information obtained when taking a patient history.

- **S**igns/symptoms—assessment findings and history as they relate to the chief complaint
  - ▶ When did it start/occur (time, sudden, gradual)? What was the child doing when it started/occurred?
  - ▶ How long did it last? Does it come and go? Is it still present?
  - ▶ Where is the problem? Describe character and severity if painful (use pain scale).
  - ▶ Radiation? Aggravating or alleviating factors?
  - ▶ Previous history of same? If yes, what was the diagnosis?
- **A**llergies—to medications, food, environmental causes (e.g., pollen), and products (e.g., latex)
- **M**edications
  - ▶ Prescription and over-the-counter medications the child is currently taking
  - ▶ Determine name of medication, dose, route, frequency and indication for the medication
- (Pertinent) **P**ast medical history
  - ▶ Is the child currently under a physician's care?
  - ▶ Serious childhood illnesses—age, complications
  - ▶ Hospitalizations—age, reason for admission, length of stay
  - ▶ Surgical procedures—age, reason for procedure, complications

- ▶ Trauma/injuries and fractures/ingestions, burns—age, circumstances surrounding event, treatment, complications
- ▶ Immunization status with regard to diphtheria, tetanus, pertussis, varicella, poliomyelitis, *haemophilus influenzae* type B, hepatitis B, rubeola, rubella, mumps, etc.
- ▶ For infants and toddlers, obtain a birth history
  - ○ Maternal age, gestational duration, prematurity, birth weight
  - ○ Complications during pregnancy or delivery (e.g., c-section, forceps delivery)
  - ○ Congenital anomalies
  - ○ "Did the baby go home with you?"
- **L**ast oral intake
  - ○ Time of last meal and fluid intake
  - ○ Changes in eating pattern or fluid intake
- ▶ For infants, determine if breast or bottle fed; if formula is used, which type; feeding difficulties
- **E**vents leading to the illness or injury
  - ▶ Onset, duration, and precipitating factors
  - ▶ Associated factors such as toxic inhalants, drugs, alcohol
  - ▶ Injury scenario and mechanism of injury
  - ▶ Treatment given by caregiver

The Emergency Nurses Association (ENA) recommends use of the CIAMPEDS mnemonic.

- **C**hief complaint
  - ▶ Reason for the child's visit to the emergency department
  - ▶ Duration of complaint

- **I**mmunizations/isolation
  - ▸ Evaluate scheduled immunizations for the child's age
  - ▸ Evaluate the child's exposure to communicable diseases (e.g., chickenpox, meningitis)
- **A**llergies to medications, food, environmental causes (e.g., pollen), products (e.g., latex), and environment
- **M**edications
  - ▸ Prescription and over-the-counter medications the child is currently taking
    - ○ Include herbal and dietary supplements
  - ▸ Determine name of medication, dose, route, frequency, and indication for each medication
- **P**ast medical history
  - ▸ Child's health status, including prior illnesses, injuries, hospitalizations, surgeries, and chronic physical and psychiatric illnesses
  - ▸ Use of alcohol, tobacco, drugs, or other substances of abuse
  - ▸ Neonate's history: prenatal and birth history, including maternal complications during pregnancy or delivery, infant's gestational age and birth weight, number of days infant remained hospitalized after delivery
  - ▸ Date and description of last menstrual period
  - ▸ For sexually active patients: include type of birth control used, barrier protection, prior treatment for sexually transmitted diseases, pregnancies (gravida) and births, miscarriages, abortions, living children (para)

- **P**arent's/caregiver's impression of the child's condition
  - ▶ Identify the patient's primary caregiver
  - ▶ Consider cultural differences that may affect the caregiver's impressions
  - ▶ Evaluate the caregiver's concerns and observations of the child's condition
- **E**vents surrounding illness or injury
  - ▶ Illness—duration, including date of onset and sequence of symptoms; treatment provided before arrival at emergency department
  - ▶ Injury—date/time of injury; mechanism of injury, including use of restraints/protective devices; suspected injuries; pre-hospital vital signs and treatment; circumstances leading to the injury, witnessed or unwitnessed
- **D**iet/diapers
  - ▶ Time of last meal and fluid intake, changes in eating pattern or fluid intake
  - ▶ For infants, determine if breast or bottle fed; if formula is used, which type; feeding difficulties
  - ▶ Special diet or dietary restrictions
  - ▶ Evaluation of child's urine and stool output
- (Associated) **S**ymptoms
  - ▶ Symptom identification and progression since onset of illness or injury

OPQRST is an acronym that may be used for evaluating pain.

- **O**nset—What were you doing when the pain started?
- **P**rovocation—What makes the pain better or worse? Coughing/deep breathing, anxiety/fear, treatment/procedure,

movement/positioning, parent/caregiver not present

- **Q**uality—What does the pain feel like? (Dull, sharp, pressure, burning, squeezing, stabbing, gnawing, shooting, throbbing)
- **R**egion/Radiation—Where is the pain? Is the pain in one area or does it move?
- **S**everity—On a scale of 0 to 10, with 0 being the least and 10 being the worst, what number would you assign your pain or discomfort?
- **T**ime—How long ago did the problem/discomfort begin? Have you ever had this pain before? When? How long did it last?

Physical Examination

The purpose of the physical examination in the Secondary Survey is to detect **non-life-threatening** conditions and provide care for those conditions or injuries. A detailed physical examination is presented here for completeness. A focused physical examination may be more appropriate, based on the patient's presentation and chief complaint.

- Inspect and palpate each of the major body areas for DCAP-BLS-TIC *(**D**eformities, **C**ontusions, **A**brasions, **P**enetrations/punctures, **B**urns, **L**acerations, **S**welling/edema, **T**enderness, **I**nstability, **C**repitus)*
- Auscultate breath and heart sounds

ONGOING ASSESSMENT

Purpose

- Reevaluate the patient's condition
- Assess the effectiveness of emergency care interventions provided
- Identify any missed injuries or conditions
- Observe subtle changes or trends in the patient's condition
- Alter emergency care interventions as needed
- The ongoing assessment should be:
  - ▶ Performed on EVERY patient
  - ▶ Performed after assuring completion of critical interventions
  - ▶ Performed after the detailed physical exam, if one is performed (In some situations, the patient's condition may preclude performance of the detailed physical exam.)
  - ▶ Repeated and documented every 5 minutes for an unstable patient
  - ▶ Repeated and documented every 15 minutes for a stable patient

■ TRIAGE IN THE EMERGENCY DEPT ■

GOALS OF TRIAGE

- Rapidly identify patients with life-threatening conditions
- Determine the most appropriate treatment area for patients coming to the emergency department
- Optimize use of resources
- Decrease congestion in emergency treatment areas
- Provide ongoing assessment of patients
- Provide information to patients and families regarding services, expected care, and waiting times

A five-level triage classification system based on patient presentation and expected resource utilization has demonstrated reliability and is reviewed here.

RESUSCITATION

A resuscitation condition requires immediate medical attention and maximum use of resources The patient presents with unstable vital functions with a high probability of death if immediate intervention is not begun to prevent additional airway, respiratory, hemodynamic, or neurologic instability; a time delay would be harmful to the patient. Highest priority is given to conditions including:

- Intubated patient
- Respiratory arrest
- Cardiopulmonary arrest

- Active seizure
- Unresponsiveness
- Multisystem injury

EMERGENT

An emergent condition is one that requires medical attention within 10 minutes and high resource utilization. The patient presents with threatened vital functions, with a potential threat to life or limb. Highest priority is given to conditions including:

- Altered mental status
- Unstable vital signs
- Severe pain or distress
- Moderate to severe respiratory distress
- Extremity injury with neurovascular compromise
- Fever in an infant <6 months of age

URGENT

An urgent condition is one that requires prompt treatment within 30 to 60 minutes. The patient presents with stable vital functions that are not likely to threaten life and requires medium resource utilization. The patient should be periodically reassessed (usually every 20 to 30 minutes) to ensure that there is no deterioration in his or her condition. Representative conditions include:

- Mild to moderate dehydration
- Mild to moderate respiratory distress
- Nonspecific chest pain
- Abdominal pain
- Moderate pain
- Nonpenetrating eye injury

SEMI-URGENT

A semi-urgent condition is one that can safely wait 1 to 2 hours to be evaluated without risk of death or further deterioration. The patient presents with stable vital functions and has a low need for resource utilization. The patient's illness or injury has a low probability of progression to more serious disease or development of complications. The patient with a semi-urgent condition should be reassessed periodically (usually every 30 to 60 minutes) to ensure there is no deterioration in his or her condition. Examples are the following:

- Simple laceration
- History of seizure (now awake and alert)
- Fever in a child 3 months to 3 years of age
- Head trauma without symptoms

NON-URGENT

A non-urgent condition is one that may safely wait 2 hours or more to be evaluated without risk of morbidity or mortality; the patient presents with stable vital functions and does not require resource utilization. The patient's illness or injury has a low probability of progression to more serious disease or development of complications. The patient with a non-urgent condition should be reassessed periodically (usually every 60 to 120 minutes) to ensure there is no deterioration in his or her condition. Examples:

- Upper respiratory infection
- Fever in a child >6 months of age
- Impetigo
- Conjunctivitis
- Isolated soft tissue injury
- Cold or flu
- Ear discomfort
- Sore throat
- Mild gastroenteritis
- Thrush
- Diaper rash

Triage Red Flags

Airway	• Apnea • Choking • Drooling • Stridor
Breathing	• Cyanosis • Grunting • Irregular respiratory pattern • Respiratory rate >60 breaths/min • Sternal retractions
Circulation	• Decreased peripheral perfusion • Decreased skin turgor • Decreased tearing • Dry tongue, mucous membranes • Heart rate <60 beats/min • Heart rate >200 beats/min • Hypotension • Hypothermia
Disability	• Altered mental status • Sunken or bulging fontanelle
Exposure/ environment	• Petechiae, purpura
Vital signs	• Fever >38.6° C (101° F) in an infant <3 months of age • Temperature >40° to 40.6° C (104° F to 105° F) at any age
History	• Decreased urine output • History of chronic illness • Return emergency department visit within 24 hours • Severe pain
Other	• Sixth sense—a subjective feeling or intuition that a child is more seriously ill than objective data indicate

From Fredrickson, JM. Triage. In: Kelly, SJ. ed. *Pediatric emergency nursing*, 2nd ed. Norwalk, CT, 1994, Appleton & Lange.

Respiratory
Conditions

RESPIRATORY CRISES

DEFINITIONS

- *Respiratory distress* is increased work of breathing (respiratory effort)
- *Respiratory failure* is a clinical condition in which there is inadequate blood oxygenation and/or ventilation to meet the metabolic demands of body tissues
- *Respiratory arrest* is the absence of breathing

RESPIRATORY DISTRESS

Respiratory distress is characterized by the presence of increased respiratory effort, rate, and work of breathing.

Causes of Respiratory Distress in Children

- Respiratory distress can result from a problem in the tracheobronchial tree, lungs, pleura, or chest wall.
- Asthma/reactive airway disease
- Aspiration
- Foreign body
- Congenital heart disease
- Infection (e.g., pneumonia, croup, epiglottitis, bronchiolitis)
- Medication or toxin exposure
- Trauma

Signs of Respiratory Distress

- Alert, irritable, anxious, restless
- Stridor
- Grunting
- Gurgling
- Audible wheezing
- Respiratory rate faster than normal for age (tachypnea)
- Increased depth of breathing (hyperpnea)
- Intercostal retractions
- Head-bobbing
- See-saw respirations (abdominal breathing)
- Nasal flaring
- Neck muscle use
- Central cyanosis that resolves with oxygen administration
- Mild tachycardia

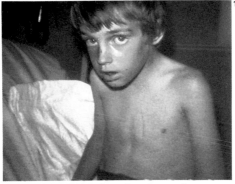

A child exhibiting signs of respiratory distress.

RESPIRATORY FAILURE

- Respiratory failure is the most common cause of cardiopulmonary arrest in children. It is often preceded by respiratory distress in which the child's work of breathing is increased in an attempt to compensate for hypoxia.
- Potential respiratory failure is based on clinical observation of signs of respiratory distress.
- Failure to improve (or deterioration) after treatment for respiratory distress indicates respiratory failure.

Causes of Respiratory Failure in Children

- Infection (e.g., croup, epiglottitis, bronchiolitis, pneumonia)
- Foreign body
- Asthma/reactive airway disease
- Smoke inhalation
- Submersion syndrome
- Pneumothorax, hemothorax

- Congenital abnormalities
- Neuromuscular disease
- Medication or toxin exposure
- Trauma
- Congestive heart failure
- Metabolic disease with acidosis

Signs of Respiratory Failure

- Sleepy, intermittently combative, or agitated
- Decreased muscle tone
- Decreased level of responsiveness or response to pain
- Inadequate respiratory rate, effort, or chest excursion
- Tachypnea with periods of bradypnea; slowing to bradypnea/agonal breathing

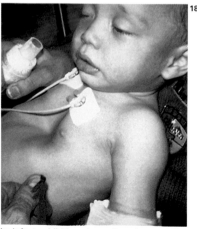

18

An infant exhibiting signs of respiratory failure.

RESPIRATORY ARREST

Signs of Respiratory Arrest

- Mottling; peripheral and central cyanosis
- Unresponsive to voice or touch
- Absent chest wall motion
- Absent respirations
- Weak to absent pulses
- Bradycardia or asystole
- Limp muscle tone

Signs of Increased Work of Breathing

VISIBLE SIGNS (LOOK)

- Anxious appearance, concentration on breathing
- Respiratory rate faster than normal for age
- Use of accessory muscles
- Leaning forward to inhale
- Inspiratory retractions
- Nasal flaring
- Head bobbing
- Seesaw (chest/abdominal) movement

AUDIBLE SIGNS (LISTEN)

• Stridor	• Grunting
• Wheezing	• Gurgling
• Crackles	• Gasping

First Impression of Respiratory Emergencies

ASSESSMENT	RESPIRATORY DISTRESS	RESPIRATORY FAILURE	RESPIRATORY ARREST
Mental status	Alert, irritable, anxious, restless	Decreased level of responsiveness or response to pain	Unresponsive to voice or touch
Muscle tone		Normal or decreased	Limp
Body position	Able to maintain sitting position (children older than 4 months) May assume tripod position	• May assume tripod position • May need support to maintain sitting position as patient tires	Unable to maintain sitting position (infant >7-9 mos)
Respiratory rate	Faster than normal for age	Tachypnea with periods of bradypnea; slowing to bradypnea/agonal breathing	Absent
Respiratory effort	• Intercostal retractions • Nasal flaring • Neck muscle use • See-saw respiratons	Inadequate respiratory effort or chest excursion	Absent
Audible airway sounds	Stridor, wheezing, gurgling	Stridor, wheezing, grunting, gasping	Absent
Skin color	Pink or pale; central cyanosis resolves with oxygen administration	Central cyanosis despite oxygen administration; mottling	Mottling; peripheral and central cyanosis

50

Immediate Interventions for Respiratory Emergencies

FIRST IMPRESSION	INTERVENTIONS
Respiratory distress	• Approach promptly, but work at a moderate pace • Permit the child to assume a position of comfort • Correct hypoxia by giving oxygen without causing agitation • Provide further interventions based on assessment findings
Respiratory failure	• Move quickly • Open the airway and suction if necessary • Correct hypoxia by giving high-flow oxygen • Begin assisted ventilation if the patient does not improve • Provide further interventions based on assessment findings
Respiratory arrest	• Move quickly • Immediately open the airway and suction if necessary • Begin ventilating with 100% oxygen • Reassess for return of spontaneous respiration • Provide further interventions based on assessment findings

Modified from: Foltin GL, Tunik MG, Cooper A, Markenson D, Treiber M, Skomorowsky A: Teaching resource for instructors in prehospital pediatrics for paramedics, New York, 2002, Center for Pediatric Emergency Medicine.

CROUP SEVERITY

- Mild croup—Normal color, normal mental status, air entry with stridor audible only with stethoscope, no retractions
- Moderate croup—Normal color, stridor audible, mild to moderate retractions, slightly diminished air entry in an anxious child
- Severe croup—Cyanosis, loud stridor, significant decrease in air entry, marked retractions in a highly anxious child

Croup score may be useful in determining the severity of airway obstruction. It is based on color, level of alertness, degree of stridor, air movement, and degree of retractions. A score of 3 necessitates hospitalization if unresponsive to therapy.

Westley Croup Score		
CRITERIA	**PRESENTATION**	**POINTS**
Retractions	None	0
	Mild	1
	Moderate	2
	Severe	3
Air entry	Normal	0
	Decreased but easily audible	1
	Severely decreased	2
Inspiratory stridor	None	0
	When agitated	1
	At rest, with stethoscope	2
	At rest, without stethoscope	4
Cyanosis	None	0
	With agitation	4
	At rest	5
Alertness (level of responsiveness)	Alert	0
	Restless, anxious	2
	Altered mental status	5
Croup score 0-1: Mild croup Croup score 2-7: Moderate croup Croup score ≥8: Severe croup		

FOREIGN BODY AIRWAY OBSTRUCTION

Description

Foreign body airway obstruction (FBAO) may be seen at any age, but children younger than 5 years of age are especially vulnerable. One third of aspirated objects are nuts, particularly peanuts. Laryngotracheal foreign bodies typically produce an acute obstruction. A foreign body in a bronchus may result in a more subtle presentation.

History

- Fewer than 50% of children will have a history of witnessed or suspected foreign body aspiration or a choking spell.
- Frequently, the child presents after a sudden episode of coughing or choking while eating, with subsequent wheezing, coughing, or stridor.

Physical Examination

- General signs and symptoms
  - ▶ Sudden onset of respiratory distress
  - ▶ Abnormal respiratory sounds, including wheezing, inspiratory stridor, or decreased breath sounds; coughing or gagging
  - ▶ Agitation
  - ▶ Cyanosis
  - ▶ Facial petechiae (may be present because of increased intrathoracic pressure)

Performance Guidelines for a Conscious Choking Infant

- Assess the infant. If the infant can cough or cry, watch him or her closely to ensure that the object is expelled. If the infant is unable to cough or cry, provide care.

- Administer back blows.
  - While supporting the infant's head and neck, place the infant over one arm, face down. Position the infant's head slightly lower than the rest of the body.
  - Using the heel of one hand, deliver up to five back blows forcefully between the infant's shoulder blades. If the foreign body is not expelled, deliver chest thrusts.

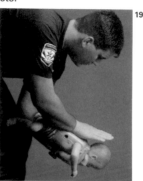

19

To clear a foreign body from a conscious infant's airway, deliver up to five back blows between the infant's shoulder blades with the heel of one hand.

- Administer chest thrusts if needed.
  - Support the infant's head and neck. Position the infant between your hands and arms and turn the infant onto his or her back.
  - Imagine a line between the nipples. Place the flat part of your middle and ring fingers about one finger-width below this imaginary line. Deliver up to five quick downward chest thrusts.

- ► Check the patient's mouth. If the foreign body is seen, remove it. Do NOT perform a blind finger sweep!

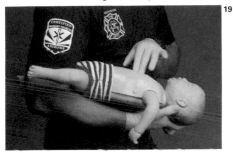

19

If back blows do not relieve the obstruction, deliver up to five chest thrusts about one finger's width below the nipple line.

- Open the airway and attempt rescue breathing.
  - ► If rescue breathing does not cause the infant's chest to rise, reposition the head and reattempt rescue breathing. If the chest does not rise (the airway remains obstructed), continue the sequence of up to five back blows, up to five chest thrusts, and breathing attempts until the object is dislodged (and expelled) and rescue breathing is successful, or the victim becomes unconscious.

Performance Guidelines for an Unconscious Choking Infant

- Place the infant in a supine position on a hard surface.
- Using a head tilt—chin lift or tongue—jaw lift (or jaw thrust without head tilt if trauma is suspected), open the airway.

- ► Check the nose and mouth for secretions, emesis, a foreign body, and other obstructions. Suction fluids and particulate matter as necessary.
- ► If a foreign body is visible, remove it using a finger sweep. Do NOT perform a blind finger sweep! Remove the foreign body only if it is visualized.
- Attempt to ventilate the infant with a bag-valve-mask device with 100% oxygen. If the chest does not rise, reposition the infant's head, reopen the airway, and try to ventilate again.
- If the chest does not rise, begin CPR.
- If basic airway maneuvers are not successful in clearing an obstructed airway:
  - ► Perform direct laryngoscopy and attempt to locate the obstruction. Remove the foreign body with pediatric Magill forceps if it is clearly visible. If removal is successful, reassess breathing and resume bag-valve-mask ventilation.
  - ► If unsuccessful, attempt tracheal intubation and ventilate the patient.
  - ► If the infant cannot be intubated, attempt bag-valve-mask ventilation.
  - ► Needle cricothyrotomy may be considered if complete airway obstruction exists and bag-valve-mask ventilation is unsuccessful (check local protocol).
  - ► Removal of the foreign body by bronchoscopy should be attempted in a controlled environment.
- If the obstruction is removed:
  - ► Assess breathing. Suction fluids and particulate matter if necessary. If the infant is not breathing, give two rescue breaths.

- ► Assess circulation and perfusion.
- ► If there is no pulse or other signs of circulation, or if the heart rate is <60 beats/min with signs of poor perfusion, begin chest compressions.
- ► If breathing is absent but a pulse is present, deliver one breath every 3 to 5 seconds (12 to 20 breaths/min) and monitor the infant's pulse.
- ► If the infant is breathing (and breathing is effective), reassess frequently.
- ► Assess mental status.
- ► Expose as necessary to perform further assessments while maintaining the infant's body temperature.
- ► Perform a focused history and detailed physical examination only if they will not interfere with lifesaving interventions.

Performance Guidelines for a Conscious Choking Child

- Assess the child's ability to speak or cough. Ask, "Are you choking?"
- If the child can cough or speak, watch closely to ensure that the object is expelled.
- If the child cannot cough or speak, perform abdominal thrusts.
  - ► Stand behind the child and wrap your arms around the child's waist.
  - ► Abdominal thrusts should be delivered two fingers width above the navel. Make a fist with one hand. Place the fist on the thrust site, with thumb side in. Place your other hand on top of the fist. Perform a quick inward and upward thrust.

▶ Continue performing abdominal thrusts until the foreign body is expelled or the child becomes unresponsive.

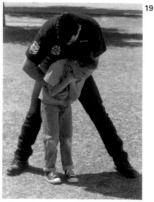

Clearing a foreign body airway obstruction in a conscious child.

Performance Guidelines for an Unconscious Choking Child

- Confirm that the patient is unresponsive.
- Place the child in a supine position on a hard surface, being sure to protect the head, neck, and spine.
- Using a head tilt—chin lift or tongue—jaw lift (or jaw thrust without head tilt if trauma is suspected), open the airway.
  - ▶ Check the nose and mouth for secretions, emesis, a foreign body, and other obstructions. Suction fluids and particulate matter as necessary.
  - ▶ If a foreign body is visible, remove it using a finger sweep. Do NOT perform a blind finger sweep! Remove the foreign body only if it is visualized.

- Attempt to ventilate the child with a bag-valve-mask device with 100% oxygen. If the chest does not rise, reposition the child's head, reopen the airway, and try again to ventilate with the bag-valve-mask.
- If the chest does not rise, begin CPR.

- If basic airway maneuvers are not successful in clearing an obstructed airway:
  - ► Perform direct laryngoscopy and attempt to locate the obstruction. Remove the foreign body with pediatric Magill forceps if it is clearly visible. If removal is successful, reassess breathing and resume bag-valve-mask ventilation.
  - ► If unsuccessful, attempt tracheal intubation and ventilate the patient.
  - ► If the child cannot be intubated, attempt bag-valve-mask ventilation.
  - ► Needle cricothyrotomy may be considered if complete airway obstruction exists and bag-valve-mask ventilation is unsuccessful (check local protocol).
  - ► Removal of the foreign body by bronchoscopy should be attempted in a controlled environment.
- If the obstruction is removed:
  - ► Assess breathing. If the child is not breathing, give two rescue breaths.
  - ► Assess circulation and perfusion.
    - ○ If there is no pulse or other signs of circulation, or if the heart rate is <60 beats/min with signs of poor perfusion, begin chest compressions.
    - ○ If breathing is absent but a pulse is present, deliver one breath every 3 to 5 seconds (12 to 20 breaths/min) and monitor the child's pulse.
  - ► If the victim is breathing (and breathing is effective):
    - ○ Turn the child to the side (recovery position) if trauma is not suspected.
    - ○ Reassess the child frequently.
  - ► Assess mental status.

- ▶ Expose as necessary to perform further assessments while maintaining the child's body temperature.
- ▶ Perform a focused history and detailed physical only if doing so will not interfere with lifesaving interventions.

RECOVERY POSITION

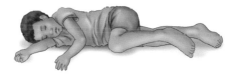

Risk Factors for Death from Asthma

- History of sudden severe exacerbations
- Prior intubation for asthma
- Prior admission for asthma to an ICU
- Two or more hospitalizations for asthma in the past year
- Three or more emergency care visits for asthma in the past year
- Hospitalization or emergency department visit for asthma in past month
- Use of more than 2 metered-dose inhaler (MDI) canisters of short-acting inhaled beta-2 agonist per month
- Serious psychiatric disease, including depression, or psychosocial problems
- Difficulty in perceiving airflow obstruction or its severity

Comparison of Upper Airway Emergencies

	CROUP	EPIGLOTTITIS	BACTERIAL TRACHEITIS	FOREIGN BODY
Age	6 months to 3 years	3 to 7 years	6 months to 3 years	<5 years most common
Cause	Viral	Bacterial	Bacterial	Food, toys, coins
Incidence	80%	8%	2%	2%
Seasonal preference	Late fall, early winter	None	None	None
Onset	Gradual	Sudden	Gradual	Sudden
Fever	Low	High	High	None
Appearance	Nontoxic	Toxic	Toxic	Varies depending on location
Posture	No preference	Upright, leaning forward, drooling	Upright	Varies depending on location
Sore throat	No	Yes	Minimal	Varies depending on location
Cry	Bark, stridor	Muffled	Bark, stridor	Varies depending on location

RESCUE BREATHING

- Rescue breathing should be performed with a mask equipped with a one-way valve or similar device. Personal protective equipment should always be readily available, including masks with one-way valves for ventilating pediatric patients.

- Deliver two breaths (1 second per breath), pausing after the first breath. The volume of air delivered should be sufficient to cause gentle chest rise. The airway is clear if air enters freely and the chest rises.

- If the child's chest does not rise during rescue breathing, ventilation is not effective.
  - ▶ If the chest doe not rise, either the airway is obstructed or more volume or pressure is needed to provide effective ventilation.
  - ▶ Readjust the position of the head, ensure the mouth is open, and reattempt to ventilate.

- Suspect a foreign body airway obstruction if the chest fails to rise despite attempts to ventilate.

SUCTIONING

Before suctioning, note the child's heart rate, oxygen saturation, and color. Monitor the child's heart rate and clinical appearance during suctioning. Bradycardia may result from stimulation of the posterior pharynx, larynx, or trachea. If bradycardia occurs or the child's clinical appearance deteriorates, interrupt suctioning and ventilate with high-concentration oxygen until the child's heart rate returns to normal.

Insertion of a suction catheter and suctioning should take no longer than 10 seconds per attempt. To suction to remove material that completely obstructs the airway, more time may be necessary.

AIRWAY ADJUNCTS

Appropriate Oropharyngeal Airway

AGE	WEIGHT (kg)	AIRWAY SIZE
Newborn/small infant (0-3 months)	3-5	Newborn
Infant (3-6 months)	6-7	Infant/small child
Infant (7-10 months)	8-9	Infant/small child
Toddler (11-18 months)	10-11	Small child
Small child (19-35 months)	12-14	Child
Child (3-4 years)	15-18	Child
Child (5-6 years)	19-22	Child/small adult
Large child (7-9 years)	24-30	Child/small adult
Adult (10-12 years)	32-40	Medium adult

Based on Broselow Resuscitation Tape

Airway Adjuncts

DEVICE	INDICATIONS	SIZING
Oropharyngeal airway (oral airway, OPA)	• To aid in maintaining an open airway in an unresponsive patient who is not intubated • To aid in maintaining an open airway in an unresponsive patient with no gag reflex that is being ventilated with a bag-valve-mask or other positive-pressure device • May be used as a bite block after insertion of a tracheal tube or orogastric tube	From corner of mouth to angle of jaw
Nasopharyngeal airway (nasal airway, NPA)	• To aid in maintaining an airway when use of an OPA is contraindicated or impossible (e.g., trismus, seizures, biting, clenched jaws or teeth) • May be useful in patients requiring frequent suctioning • Dental or oral trauma	From tip of nose to angle of jaw or tip of ear
Laryngeal mask airway (LMA)	• Patient for whom intubation has been unsuccessful and ventilation is difficult • Patient for whom airway management is necessary but healthcare provider is untrained in technique of visualized orotracheal intubation • Many elective surgical procedures	Because masks are available in several sizes, LMA can be used for patients of all ages, from neonates to adults

65

Oxygen Percentage Delivery

DEVICE	APPROXIMATE INSPIRED OXYGEN CONCENTRATION	LITER FLOW (L/minute)
Nasal cannula	Up to 50%	1-6
Simple face mask	35%-60%	6-10
Partial rebreather mask	50%-60%	10-12
Nonrebreather mask	60%-95%	10-15
Face tent	35%-40%	10-15
Oxygen hood	80%-90%	10-15
Blow-by (via face mask)	30%-40%	10

BAG-VALVE-MASK VENTILATION

To ensure proper timing when ventilating an infant or child, use the mnemonic "squeeze, release, release." Say, "squeeze" when ventilating with the bag. Release the bag as soon as chest rise is visible and say, "release, release" to ensure adequate time for exhalation.

TRACHEAL INTUBATION

INDICATIONS

Blind nasotracheal intubation is contraindicated until age 10 years.

- Hypoxemia despite supplemental oxygen
- Inadequate ventilation with less invasive methods
- Actual or potential decrease in airway protective reflexes (e.g., drug overdose, head trauma)
- Respiratory failure or arrest, gasping or agonal respirations
- Present or impending airway obstruction (e.g., stridor, significant increase in work of

breathing, inhalation injury, epiglottitis, bleeding in the airway, asthma, severe pulmonary edema)

- Meconium aspiration during delivery
- Unstable chest wall, inadequate respiratory muscle function, or severe chest trauma (e.g., severe flail chest, pulmonary contusion, pneumothorax)
- When mechanical ventilatory support is anticipated (e.g., acute respiratory failure, chest trauma, increased work of breathing, shock, increased intracranial pressure)

TWELVE STEPS OF PEDIATRIC TRACHEAL INTUBATION[1]

1. Oxygenate and ventilate the patient
2. Prepare the equipment
3. Position the patient
4. Provide suctioning and oxygenation
5. Open the patient's mouth
6. Control the patient's tongue
7. Control the patient's epiglottis
8. Locate landmarks for intubation
9. Insert the tracheal tube
10. Confirm correct placement
11. Secure the tube in place
12. Resume oxygenation and ventilation

TROUBLESHOOTING (DOPE)

- **D**isplaced tube (e.g., right mainstem or esophageal intubation)—Reassess tube position
- **O**bstructed tube (e.g., blood or secretions are obstructing air flow)—Suction
- **P**neumothorax (tension)—Needle thoracostomy
- **E**quipment problem/failure—Check equipment and oxygen source

Appropriate Resuscitation Bag and Oxygen Mask Size

AGE	WEIGHT (kg)	RESUSCITATION BAG	OXYGEN MASK
Newborn/small infant (0-3 months)	3-5	Infant	Newborn
Infant (3-6 months)	6-7	Child	Newborn
Infant (7-10 months)	8-9	Child	Newborn/pediatric
Toddler (11-18 months)	10-11	Child	Pediatric
Small child (19-35 months)	12-14	Child	Pediatric
Child (3-4 years)	15-18	Child	Pediatric
Child (5-6 years)	19-22	Child	Pediatric
Large child (7-9 years)	24-30	Child/adult	Adult
Adult (10-12 years)	32-40	Adult	Adult

Based on Broselow Resuscitation Tape

INDICATIONS

- Excessive work of breathing, which may lead to fatigue and respiratory failure
- Loss of protective airway reflexes (e.g., cough, gag)
- Combative patients requiring airway control
- Uncontrolled seizure activity (to provide airway control)
- Functional or anatomic airway obstruction
- Head trauma and Glasgow Coma Score <8
- Severe asthma
- Inadequate central nervous system control of ventilation
- Need for high peak inspiratory pressure or positive end-expiratory pressure to maintain effective alveolar gas exchange
- To permit sedation for diagnostic studies while ensuring airway protection and control of secretions

7 Ps OF RAPID SEQUENCE INTUBATION (RSI)

- **P**reparation (zero minus 10 minutes)
- **P**reoxygenate (zero minus 5 minutes)
- **P**remedicate (zero minus 3 minutes)
- **P**aralysis with sedation (zero)
- **P**rotect the airway (zero + 15 seconds)
- **P**ass the tube and proof of placement (zero + 45 seconds)
- **P**ost-intubation management (zero + 60 seconds)

Equipment Selection for Pediatric Tracheal Intubation

AGE	WEIGHT (kg)	BLADE SIZE	BLADE TYPE	TRACHEAL TUBE SIZE (mm)	TRACHEAL TUBE CUFF	TRACHEAL TUBE LENGTH (cm at lip)	STYLET (F)
Newborn/small infant (0-3 months)	3-5	0-1	Straight	2.5-3.5†	Uncuffed	10-10.5	6
Infant (3-6 months)	6-7	1	Straight	3.5	Uncuffed	10-10.5	6
Infant (7-10 months)	8-9	1	Straight	3.5-4.0	Uncuffed	10.5-12	6
Toddler (11-18 months)	10-11	1	Straight	4	Uncuffed	11-12	6
Small child (19-35 months)	12-14	2	Straight	4.5	Uncuffed	12.5-13.5	6
Child (3-4 years)	15-18	2	Straight or curved	5	Uncuffed	14-15	6
Child (5-6 years)	19-22	2	Straight or curved	5.5	Uncuffed	15.5-16.5	14
Large child (7-9 years)	24-30	2-3	Straight or curved	6	Cuffed	17-18	14
Adult (10-12 years)	32-40	3	Straight or curved	6.5	Cuffed	18.5-19.5	14

Based on Broselow Resuscitation Tape   †Use 2.5 for premature infant. Use 3.0-3.5 for term infant.

CONTRAINDICATIONS

Absolute Contraindications

Before initiating RSI, the individual performing the procedure must be trained, appropriately credentialed, and prepared to perform a cricothyrotomy in the event of a failed airway.

- Patients in whom alternative airway control (i.e., cricothyrotomy) would be difficult or impossible due to anatomy or massive neck swelling
- Patients who would be difficult or impossible to intubate after paralysis
- Operator unfamiliarity with the medications used for the RSI procedure

Relative Contraindications

The risk of complications must be compared to the benefit of obtaining airway control.

- Severely increased intracranial pressure
- Known hypersensitivity to the medications used for the procedure
- Known unstable cervical spine injury or fracture

NEEDLE CRICOTHYROTOMY

DESCRIPTION

- Needle cricothyrotomy (also called percutaneous cricothyrotomy) is a method of providing ventilation by insertion of a large bore over-the-needle catheter into the cricothyroid membrane. This procedure may be indicated in cases of upper airway obstruction that cannot be relieved by less invasive methods such as head positioning, suctioning, foreign body airway maneuvers, bag-valve-mask ventilation, and tracheal intubation.

- Needle cricothyrotomy can be extremely difficult to perform in infants and young children because of the mobility of the larynx and trachea and the softness of the laryngeal cartilage in these patients, making palpation of the landmarks for the procedure difficult and collapse of the upper airway with labored breathing more likely.[2] This procedure requires special training and frequent refresher training to maintain skill proficiency.

INDICATIONS

- Conditions in which intubation is difficult or impossible
- Craniofacial abnormalities
- Congenital laryngeal anomalies
- Excessive oropharyngeal hemorrhage
- Massive traumatic or congenital deformities
- Complete upper airway obstruction
- Laryngeal fracture
- Pharyngeal/laryngeal burns
- Subglottic stenosis
- Respiratory arrest or near arrest in patients who cannot be intubated tracheally
- Cervical spine fracture with respiratory compromise in patients who cannot be tracheally intubated

CONTRAINDICATIONS

Unavailable or inadequate equipment

Sedative Options during Rapid Sequence Intubation

CLINICAL CONDITION	BLOOD PRESSURE	ADJUNCTIVE AGENT	SEDATIVE
Status asthmaticus	N/A	Atropine*	Ketamine *OR* midazolam
Head injury or increased ICP	Normal	Lidocaine	Etomidate *OR* thiopental *OR* midazolam
	Decreased	Lidocaine	Etomidate *OR* thiopental (low-dose) *OR* midazolam
Status epilepticus	N/A		Thiopental *OR* midazolam *OR* propofol†
Shock	Mild	Atropine (if ketamine used)	Etomidate (low dose) *OR* ketamine *OR* midazolam (low dose)
	Severe	Atropine (if ketamine used)	Etomidate (low dose) *OR* ketamine *OR* none
No head injury or increased ICP	Normal	Atropine (if ketamine used)	Etomidate *OR* thiopental *OR* midazolam *OR* ketamine *OR* propofol
	Decreased	Atropine (if ketamine used)	Etomidate *OR* midazolam (low dose) *OR* ketamine

*Atropine administration should be standard for all children younger than 1 year of age; children who are bradycardic; children younger than 5 years of age who are to receive succinylcholine; and adolescents who receive a second dose of succinylcholine. Atropine is suggested if ketamine is used.

†Use with caution in critically ill or injured children.

73

SURGICAL CRICOTHYROTOMY

DESCRIPTION

- A surgical cricothyrotomy is the creation of an opening into the cricothyroid membrane with a scalpel to allow rapid entrance to the airway for temporary oxygenation and ventilation. This procedure may be indicated in cases of upper airway obstruction that cannot be relieved by less invasive methods such as head positioning, suctioning, foreign body airway maneuvers, bag-valve-mask ventilation, and tracheal intubation.

- Surgical cricothyrotomy can be difficult to perform in infants and young children because of the difficulty in palpating and identifying the important landmarks of the neck. For that reason and because of the small diameter of the cricoid cartilage, the procedure is not recommended in children under the age of 10.[3] This procedure requires special training and frequent refresher training to maintain skill proficiency.

INDICATIONS

Surgical cricothyrotomy is rarely indicated for the infant or young child. If the procedure is absolutely necessary, the most experienced person available, preferably an experienced surgeon, should perform it.

- Conditions in which intubation is difficult or impossible
- Craniofacial abnormalities
- Congenital laryngeal anomalies
- Excessive oropharyngeal hemorrhage
- Massive traumatic or congenital deformities

- Complete upper airway obstruction
- Laryngeal fracture
- Pharyngeal/laryngeal burns
- Subglottic stenosis
- Respiratory arrest or near arrest in patients who cannot be intubated tracheally
- Cervical spine fracture with respiratory compromise in patients who cannot be intubated tracheally

CONTRAINDICATIONS

- Children under the age of 10 years
- Adequate nonsurgical airway
- Unavailable or inadequate equipment
- Bleeding diatheses

NEEDLE THORACOSTOMY

DESCRIPTION

Needle thoracostomy (also called needle decompression) is the insertion of an over-the-needle catheter into the chest to relieve a tension pneumothorax. The procedure converts a tension pneumothorax to a simple, open pneumothorax.

INDICATIONS

Suspected tension pneumothorax as evidenced by:

- Progressively worsening dyspnea
- Tachypnea
- Tachycardia
- Poor ventilation despite an open airway
- Restlessness and agitation
- Increased airway resistance when patient is ventilated (poor bag compliance)

- Hyperresonance to percussion on the affected side
- Diminished or absent breath sounds on the affected side
- Decreased level of responsiveness
- Hypotension
- Tracheal deviation away from side of injury (may or may not be present)
- Distended neck veins (may not be present if hypovolemia is present or hypotension is severe)
- Cyanosis

CONTRAINDICATIONS

There are no contraindications to this procedure if the patient's clinical presentation, history, and physical findings suggest the presence of a tension pneumothorax.

CARDIAC CONDITIONS

CHAIN OF SURVIVAL

The pediatric chain of survival represents a sequential series of events to assess, support, or restore effective ventilation and circulation to the infant or child experiencing a respiratory or cardiorespiratory arrest. The sequence consists of four important steps.

- Prevention of illness or injury
- Early cardiopulmonary resuscitation (CPR)
- Early emergency medical services (EMS) activation
- Early advanced life support (ALS)

THE PEDIATRIC CHAIN OF SURVIVAL[19]

Activating EMS is delayed until after a trial of early CPR. This is based on the higher likelihood of respiratory conditions and lower likelihood of ventricular fibrillation as the cause of cardiopulmonary arrest in the pediatric patient.

■ PEDIATRIC AGE CLASSIFICATIONS ■

- Newly born: neonate in the first minutes to hours following birth
- Neonate: Birth to 1 month
- Infant: 1 to 12 months of age
- Toddler: 1 to 3 years of age
- Preschooler: 4 to 5 years of age
- School age: 6 to 12 years of age
- Adolescent: The period between the end of childhood (beginning of puberty) and adulthood (18 years of age)

STAGES OF CARDIAC CYCLE[25]

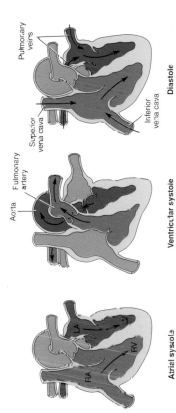

Atrial sysgole

Ventricular systole

Diastole

A. Atrial systole. The atria contract and force blood into the relaxed ventricles.
B. Ventricular systole. The ventricles contract, forcing blood into the pulmonary artery and aorta.
C. Diastole. Both atria and ventricles are relaxed and fill with blood.

First Impression of Cardiovascular Emergencies

ASSESSMENT	IMMINENT CARDIOPULMONARY FAILURE	CARDIOPULMONARY FAILURE	CARDIOPULMONARY ARREST
Mental status	Alert, irritable, anxious, restless	Sleepy, intermittently combative, or agitated	Unresponsive to voice or touch
Muscle tone	Normal or decreased	Normal or decreased	Limp
Body position	Able to maintain sitting position (children older than 4 months) May assume tripod position	• May assume tripod position • May need help maintaining sitting position as patient tires	Unable to maintain sitting position (> 4 months)
Respiratory rate	Faster than normal for age	Tachypnea with periods of bradypnea; slowing to bradypnea/agonal breathing	Absent
Respiratory effort	• Intercostal retractions • Nasal flaring • Neck muscle use • See-saw respiratons	• Nasal flaring; see-saw respirations • Increased respiratory effort at sternal notch • Marked use of accessory muscles • Retractions, head bobbing • Inadequate chest excursion	Absent
Audible airway sounds	Stridor, wheezing, gurgling	Stridor, wheezing, grunting, gasping	Absent
Skin color	Pink or pale; central cyanosis resolves with O₂	Central cyanosis despite O₂; mottling	Mottling; peripheral and central cyanosis

Immediate Interventions for Cardiovascular Emergencies

FIRST IMPRESSION	INTERVENTIONS
Imminent cardiopulmonary failure	• Approach promptly, but work at a moderate pace • Permit child to assume a position of comfort • Correct hypoxia by giving oxygen without causing agitation • Provide further interventions based on assessment findings
Cardiopulmonary failure	• Move quickly • Open airway and suction if necessary • Correct hypoxia by giving high-flow oxygen • Begin assisted ventilation if patient does not improve • Provide further interventions based on assessment findings
Cardiopulmonary arrest	• Move quickly • Immediately open the airway and suction if necessary • Use positioning or adjuncts as necessary • Provide assisted ventilation with high-concentration oxygen • Perform chest compressions as necessary • Apply cardiac monitor and determine cardiac rhythm • Perform endotracheal intubation if assisted ventilation is ineffective or if airway cannot otherwise be maintained • Administer fluids, medications, or defibrillation as indicated • Reassess for return of spontaneous respiration and circulation • Provide further interventions based on assessment findings

Focused History—Cardiovascular Conditions

In addition to the SAMPLE history, consider the following questions when obtaining a focused history for a condition affecting the cardiovascular system. This list will require modification on the basis of the patient's age and chief complaint.

Shock

- History of trauma?
- Recent vomiting or diarrhea? Number of diaper changes or trips to the bathroom?
- Will the child drink?
- Has the child had a fever? For how long?
- Associated symptoms (e.g., change in mental status, shortness of breath, feeling faint, dizziness)
- History of severe asthma or allergic reactions? Previous treatment?
- Previous hospitalization for allergic reaction?
- Possible bite or sting or ingestion of nuts, shellfish, eggs? New medication?

Dysrhythmias

- When did it start or occur (time, sudden, gradual)?
- What was the child doing when it started or occurred?
- How long did it last? Does it come and go? Is it still present?
- Does anything make the symptoms better or worse (e.g., change in position, rest)?
- Associated symptoms (e.g., palpitations, change in mental status, shortness of breath, feeling faint, dizziness)

- Previous hospitalization for heart-related problem?

Chest pain

- When did it start or occur (time, sudden, gradual)?
- What was the child doing when it started or occurred?
- Quality (e.g., crushing, tight, stabbing, burning, squeezing)
- How long did it last? Does it come and go? Is it still present?
- Where is the problem? Describe the character and severity if pain is present (use pain scale in Chapter 5 p. 125).
- Associated symptoms (e.g., shortness of breath, feeling faint, dizziness)
- Previous history of a similar episode? If yes, what was the diagnosis?
- Does anything make the symptoms better or worse (e.g., change in position)?

Congestive heart failure

- When did it start or occur (time, sudden, gradual)?
- When was the child last well (i.e., without current symptoms)?
- History of congenital heart disease?
- Poor feeding? Recent weight gain? Decrease in activity?
- Does anything make the symptoms better or worse (e.g., lying down worsens symptoms)?

Normal Heart Rates

AGE	BEATS PER MINUTE*
Infant (1-12 months)	100-160
Toddler (1-3 years)	90-150
Preschooler (4-5 years)	80-140
School-age (6-12 years)	70-120
Adolescent (13-18 years)	60-100

*Pulse rates for a sleeping child may be 10% lower than the low rate listed in age group.

Lower Limit of Normal Systolic Blood Pressure

AGE	LOWER LIMIT OF NORMAL SYSTOLIC BLOOD PRESSURE
Term neonate (0 to 28 days)	>60 mm Hg or strong central pulse
Infant (1 to 12 months)	>70 mm Hg or strong central pulse
Child 1 to 10 years	>70 + (2 × age in years)
Child ≥ 10 years	>90 mm Hg

Average Circulating Blood Volume[11]

AGE	NORMAL BLOOD VOLUME (average)
Preterm infant	90-105 mL/kg
Term newborn	85 mL/kg
Infant >1 month to 11 months	75 mL/kg
Beyond 1 year	67-75 mL/kg
Adult	55-75 mL/kg

Response to Fluid and Blood Loss in the Pediatric Patient

	CLASS I	CLASS II	CLASS III	CLASS IV
Stage of shock		Compensated	Decompensated	Irreversible
% Blood volume loss	Up to 15%	15% to 30%	30% to 45%	>45%
Mental status	Slightly anxious	Mildly anxious; restless	Altered; lethargic; apathetic; decreased pain response	Extremely lethargic; unresponsive
Muscle tone	Normal	Normal	Normal to decreased	Limp
Respiratory rate/effort	Normal	Mild tachypnea	Moderate tachypnea	Severe tachypnea to agonal
Skin color (extremities)	Pink	Pale, mottled	Pale, mottled, mild peripheral cyanosis	Pale, mottled, central and peripheral cyanosis
Skin temperature	Cool	Cool	Cool to cold	Cold
Capillary refill	Normal	Poor (>2 sec)	Delayed (<3 sec)	Prolonged (>5 sec)
Heart rate	Usually normal if volume loss gradual; increased if loss of volume sudden	Mild tachycardia	Significant tachycardia; possible dysrhythmias; peripheral pulse weak, thready, or absent	Marked tachycardia to bradycardia (preterminal event)
Blood pressure	Normal	Lower range of normal	Decreased	Severe hypotension
Pulse pressure	Normal or increased	Narrowed	Decreased	Decreased
Urine output	Normal; concentrated	Decreased	Minimal	Minimal to absent

SHOCK

Perform an initial assessment (see Initial Assessment A)

↓

If **no** signs of congestive heart failure are present:

- Give a bolus of isotonic crystalloid solution (NS or LR) IV/IO as rapidly as needed (<20 minutes) to maintain circulating blood volume
- Check glucose. Treat if <60 mg/dL
- Maintain normal body temperature
- Correct electrolyte and acid-base disturbances

↓

Assess response (i.e., mental status, capillary refill, heart rate, respiratory effort, blood pressure)

↓

If inadequate response:

→

Hypovolemic

Hypovolemic Shock—Nontraumatic: Administer 1 or 2 additional fluid boluses as indicated. Reassess. Consider vasopressors if poor perfusion persists despite adequate ventilation, oxygenation, and volume expansion.

Hemorrhagic Shock: Administer 1 or 2 additional fluid boluses as indicated and reassess; administer packed red blood cells if available. Type and cross emergently if the child has severe trauma and life-threatening blood loss. Consider giving O-negative blood without crossmatch. Order a consult with trauma service as soon as possible.

Cardiogenic

- Consider giving a small IV/IO fluid bolus of isotonic crystalloid solution. Repeat the primary survey after each fluid bolus. The fluid bolus may be repeated on the basis of the child's response. If the child fails to improve, consider giving an inotrope (e.g., dopamine, dobutamine, or epinephrine) to improve myocardial contractility and increase cardiac output.
- Treat dysrhythmias if present and contributing to shock. Consult cardiologist for additional orders.

Distributive	**Anaphylaxis**	• Remove/discontinue the causative agent. Give epinephrine • Give 1 or 2 additional fluid boluses as indicated. Reassess. Consider inhaled bronchodilator (albuterol), diphenhydramine, methylprednisolone • Give epinephrine IV infusion for signs of decompensated shock
	Septic	• Administer 1 or 2 additional fluid boluses as indicated. Reassess • Administer a vasopressor by IV infusion for signs of decompensated shock • Give IV antibiotics
	Neurogenic	• Administer 1 or 2 additional fluid boluses as indicated. Reassess
Obstructive	**Tension pneumothorax**	• Perform needle decompression followed by chest tube insertion. Reassess
	Cardiac tamponade	• Administer 1 or 2 additional fluid boluses as indicated. Reassess • Pericardiocentesis is the definitive treatment for cardiac tamponade

CARDIOPULMONARY FAILURE

Cardiopulmonary failure is a clinical condition identified by deficits in oxygenation, ventilation, and perfusion. Respiratory failure associated with decompensated shock leads to inadequate oxygenation, ventilation, and perfusion, resulting in cardiopulmonary failure. Without prompt recognition and management, cardiopulmonary failure will deteriorate to cardiopulmonary arrest.

SIGNS

- Bradypnea with irregular, ineffective respirations
- Decreasing work of breathing (tiring)
- Capillary refill time, longer than 5 seconds
- Bradycardia
- Weak central and absent peripheral pulses
- Cool extremities
- Mottled or cyanotic skin
- Diminished level of responsiveness

CARDIOPULMONARY ARREST

Cardiac arrest is the cessation of cardiac mechanical activity, confirmed by the absence of a detectable pulse, unresponsiveness, and apnea or agonal, gasping respirations. In adults, sudden nontraumatic cardiopulmonary arrests are usually the result of underlying cardiac disease. In children, it is usually the result of respiratory failure or shock that progresses to cardiopulmonary failure with profound hypoxemia and acidosis, and eventually to cardiopulmonary arrest. The cause of cardiopulmonary arrest also varies with age, the underlying health of the child, and the location of the event.

CAUSES OF PULSELESS ELECTRICAL ACTIVITY (PEA): 4 Hs AND 4 Ts

- **H**ypovolemia
- **H**ypoxemia
- **H**ypothermia
- **H**yperkalemia

- **T**ension pneumothorax
- **T**hrombosis: lungs (massive pulmonary embolism)
- **T**ablets/toxins: drug overdose
- **T**amponade, cardiac

Major Causes of Pediatric Cardiac Arrest

Cardiovascular

- Hypovolemic shock
- Congenital heart defect
- Dysrhythmias
- Pericardial effusion
- Septic shock
- Cardiogenic shock
- Myocarditis

Respiratory

- Croup/epiglottitis
- Angioedema
- Pneumonia
- Drowning
- Bronchiolitis
- Foreign body obstruction
- Severe asthma
- Respiratory failure
- Inhalation injury
- Bronchopulmonary dysplasia

Neurologic

- CNS infection
- Ventriculoperitoneal shunt obstruction
- Botulism
- Status epilepticus

Trauma

- Head trauma
- Burns
- Hypovolemic shock
- Chest trauma

Other

- Sudden Infant Death Syndrome (SIDS)
- Metabolic disorders
- Drug toxicity
- Poisoning

From Bernstein, D: History and physical examination. In Behrman RE, Kliegman RM, Jenson HB, editors: Nelson textbook of pediatrics, ed 16, Philadelphia, 2000, Saunders.

TACHYCARDIA

Perform an initial assessment
Ensure effective oxygenation and ventilation
If pulseless, begin CPR — go to pulseless
Attach monitor/defibrillator

Narrow QRS <0.08 seconds

Probable Sinus Tachycardia or SVT

Probable sinus tachycardia:

- History explains rapid rate
- P waves present/normal
- Rhythm onset—gradual
- Ventricular rate/regularity varies with activity/stimulation
- Variable RR with constant PR
- Rate usually <220 beats/min in infant and <180 beats/min in child

Identify and treat underlying cause

Probable supraventricular tachycardia (SVT):

- History does not explain rapid rate
- P waves absent/abnormal
- Rhythm onset—abrupt
- Ventricular rate/regularity constant with activity/stimulation
- Abrupt rate changes
- Rate usually >220 beats/min or more in infant and >180 beats/min or more in child

Sick or not sick?

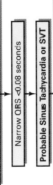

91

TACHYCARDIA

Probable Supraventricular Tachycardia **(SVT)**

Sick or not sick?

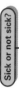

Sick (unstable)

- Consider vagal maneuvers
- If IV/IO in place, consider adenosine
- Sedate if possible, then synchronized cardioversion with 0.5 to 1.0 J/kg; increase to 2J/kg if rhythm persists

Not Sick (stable)

- Obtain 12-lead ECG
- Consult pediatric cardiologist
- Try vagal maneuvers
- Start IV
- Identify/treat causes
- Give adenosine IV
- If rhythm persists, consider amiodarone or procainamide

TACHYCARDIA
Probable Ventricular Tachycardia (**VT**)
(Wide QRS >0.08 sec)

Sick or not sick?

Sick (unstable)
- If IV/IO in place, consider adenosine
- Sedate if possible, then synchronized cardioversion with 0.5 to 1.0 J/kg; increase to 2 J/kg if rhythm persists
- Consider amiodarone or procainamide before third shock

Not Sick (stable)
- Obtain 12-lead ECG
- Consult pediatric cardiologist
- Start IV
- Identify/treat causes
- Give amiodarone slowly IV

BRADYCARDIA

Perform an initial assessment
Ensure effective oxygenation and ventilation
If pulseless, begin CPR—go to pulseless
Attach pulse oximeter and monitor/defibrillator

Not Sick (stable)

- Observe
- Support ABCs
- Consider transfer or transport to advanced life support facility

Sick (unstable)

If the bradycardia is causing severe cardiopulmonary compromise (poor perfusion, hypotension, respiratory difficulty, altered mental status):

If the heart rate is <60/min and poor systemic perfusion is present despite oxygenation and ventilation:

- Start chest compressions
- Start IV
- Give epinephrine
- Give atropine (if increased vagal tone or primary AV block)
- Consider causes
- Consider pacing

- Start IV
- Give epinephrine
- Give atropine (if increased vagal tone or primary AV block)
- Consider causes
- Consider pacing

Identify and treat possible causes
- Hypoxemia: give oxygen
- Hypothermia: use simple warming techniques
- Head injury: provide oxygenation and ventilation
- Heart block: consider atropine, chronotropic drugs, early pacing; consult pediatric cardiologist
- Heart transplant (special situation): may require pacing or large doses of sympathomimetics
- Toxins/poisons/drugs: may require antidote
- Increased vagal tone, AV block: give atropine

PULSELESS ARREST—VF/VT

Perform an initial assessment
Ensure effective oxygenation and ventilation
Perform CPR until arrival of monitor/defibrillator
Attach monitor/defibrillator and assess ECG rhythm. If VF/VT:

↓

- Shock x 1 with 2 J/kg
- Resume CPR for about 2 min
- Without interrupting CPR, start IV/IO (if not already done)
- During CPR, give vasopressor (epinephrine)

→

Assess ECG rhythm. If shockable:
- Shock x 1 with 4 J/kg
- Resume CPR for about 2 min
- During CPR, consider antiarrhythmic
- Consider reversible causes of arrest

→

Assess ECG rhythm. If shockable:

- Shock x 1 with 4 J/kg, resume CPR, give epinephrine

Electrical activities present?

- Check pulse
- If no pulse or asystole, resume CPR for about 2 min
- During CPR, give vasopressor

Pulse present?

- Assess vital signs, begin postresuscitation care

Identify and treat possible causes:

- **Hypoxemia:** give oxygen
- **Hypovolemia:** replace volume
- **Hypothermia:** use simple warming techniques
- **Hyper/hypokalemia and metabolic disorders:** correct electrolyte and acid-base disturbances
- **Tamponade:** pericardiocentesis
- **Tension pneumothorax:** needle decompression
- **Toxins/poisons/drugs:** antidote/specific therapy
- **Thromboembolism**

PULSELESS ARREST—PEA/Asystole

- Perform an initial assessment
- Ensure effective oxygenation and ventilation
- Perform CPR until arrival of monitor/defibrillator
- Attach monitor/defibrillator and assess ECG rhythm

- If asystole, confirm rhythm in a second lead
- Attempt to identify and treat underlying cause
- Resume CPR for about 2 min
- Consider placement of advanced airway, confirm tube position
- Without interrupting CPR, establish vascular access; give epinephrine every 3-5 minutes

- Resume CPR for about 2 min
- During CPR, give vasopressor

Reassess
- ECG rhythm
- Advanced airway position
- Electrode position and contact
- Effectiveness of CPR
- Proper functioning of equipment in use
- Confirm appropriate interventions
- Consider alternative medications and special resuscitation circumstances

Identify and treat possible causes:

- **H**ypoxemia: give oxygen
- **H**ypovolemia: replace volume
- **H**ypothermia: use simple warming techniques
- **H**yper/hypokalemia and metabolic disorders: correct electrolyte and acid-base disturbances
- **T**amponade: pericardiocentesis
- **T**ension pneumothorax: needle decompression
- **T**oxins/poisons/drugs: antidote/specific therapy
- **T**hromboembolism

Differential Diagnosis of Chest Pain in Pediatric Patients[16]

Musculoskeletal causes (common)

- Trauma (accidental, abuse)
- Exercise, overuse injury (strain, bursitis)
- Costochondritis (Tietze's syndrome)
- Herpes zoster (cutaneous)
- Pleurodynia
- Fibrositis
- Slipping rib
- Sickle cell anemia vaso-occlusive crisis
- Osteomyelitis (rare)
- Primary or metastatic tumor (rare)

Pulmonary causes (common)

- Pneumonia
- Pleurisy
- Asthma
- Chronic cough
- Pneumothorax
- Infarction (sickle cell anemia)
- Foreign body
- Embolism (rare)
- Pulmonary hypertension (rare)
- Tumor (rare)

Idiopathic causes (common)

- Anxiety, hyperventilation
- Panic disorder

Gastrointestinal causes (less common)

- Esophagitis (gastroesophageal reflux)
- Esophageal foreign body
- Esophageal spasm
- Cholecystitis
- Subdiaphragmatic abscess
- Perihepatitis (Fitz-Hugh-Curtis syndrome)
- Peptic ulcer disease

Cardiac causes (less common)

- Pericarditis
- Postpericardiotomy syndrome
- Endocarditis
- Mitral valve prolapse
- Aortic or subaortic stenosis
- Arrhythmias
- Marfan's syndrome (dissecting aortic aneurysm)
- Anomalous coronary artery
- Kawasaki's disease
- Cocaine, sympathomimetic ingestion
- Angina (familial hypercholesterolemia)

Other causes (less common)

- Spinal cord or nerve root compression
- Breast-related pathologic condition
- Castleman's disease (lymph node neoplasm)

BASIC LIFE SUPPORT (BLS) SKILL COMPONENTS:

- Assess/alert/attend
- Assess responsiveness
- Position the victim
- Airway
- Breathing
- Circulation/chest compressions

Assess

- Assess the scene for safety. Is it safe to approach the victim? If the scene is not safe, alert EMS for help and make sure other bystanders are aware of existing danger.
- Assess the victim for life threatening conditions and shout for help if necessary. For example, "I need help here!"
- Assess and make a quick determination regarding the nature of the emergency and the approximate age of the victim.

Alert

- Alert EMS for assistance if necessary.

Attend

Attend to the victim(s) and provide necessary care until advanced medical help (EMS) arrives and takes over.

Assess Responsiveness

- Quickly assess the child's level of responsiveness by tapping the child and speaking loudly, "Are you OK?"
  - ▶ If head or neck trauma is suspected, do not shake the child; avoid spinal injury.
- If the child is unresponsive but breathing, call EMS to facilitate transport of the child as rapidly as possible to an appropriate facility.
- The child with respiratory distress should be permitted to remain in the position he or she finds most comfortable in order to maintain patency of the partially obstructed airway.

Position the Victim

- Positioning or moving a victim may be necessary if:
  - ▶ You find an unresponsive victim lying face down
  - ▶ You must momentarily leave a breathing victim unattended
  - ▶ Victim is breathing but unresponsive
  - ▶ The victim is vomiting or has debris in his or her mouth
  - ▶ The victim's life is in immediate danger in his or her current location
- If the child is breathing and trauma to the head or neck is not suspected, place the child in the recovery position.

- Kneel at the child's waist.
- Position the child's arm that is closest to you up and away from the child's side.
- Bend the leg that is opposite you upward.
- Grasp the child's hip and shoulder and roll him or her toward you, resting the child's head on his or her extended arm. The child's bent leg should help keep him or her from rolling.
- If the child is to be left in this position for an extended period, alternate the child's position to the opposite side every 30 minutes. Continue to monitor airway, breathing, and circulation.

A = Airway

The tongue is the most common cause of airway obstruction in the unresponsive pediatric victim. Because the tongue is attached to the lower jaw, displacing the jaw forward lifts the tongue away from the back of the throat, opening the airway.

- Kneel beside the victim.
- Place one hand on the child's forehead. Place the fingers of your other hand on the bony part of the child's chin. Tilt the child's head back and open the mouth (head tilt—chin lift maneuver).
- If you suspect a neck or spinal injury, lift the child's jaw without tilting the head (jaw thrust without head tilt maneuver).

B = Breathing

- Determine if the infant or child is breathing (assess for no more than 10 seconds).
  - LOOK for rise and fall of the chest and abdomen.
  - LISTEN for exhaled air.
  - FEEL for exhaled air.

- If the patient is breathing, maintain a patent airway.
- If the patient is not breathing or if breathing is inadequate:
  - ▸ Remove any obvious airway obstruction.
  - ▸ Begin rescue breathing while maintaining a patent airway with a chin-lift or jaw thrust without head-tilt.
  - ▸ Deliver two breaths (1 second per breath) with sufficient volume to cause gentle chest rise. Allow for exhalation between breaths.

C = Circulation

- Check for a pulse for up to 10 seconds.
- In infants, assess the brachial pulse.
  - ▸ Place your thumb on the outside of the infant's arm and your index and middle fingers on the inside of the upper arm between the elbow and the shoulder.
  - ▸ Press gently and assess for a pulse for up to 10 seconds.
- Assess the carotid pulse in children over the age of 1 year.
  - ▸ Locate the thyroid cartilage (Adam's apple) with 2 to 3 fingers of one hand.
  - ▸ Using the side of the patient's neck closest to you, slide your fingers into the groove between the trachea and the sternocleidomastoid muscles and gently palpate the carotid artery. Assess for a pulse for up to 10 seconds.
- If a pulse is present but the infant or child is not breathing, give rescue breaths at a rate of 1 breath every 3 to 5 seconds (12 to 20/minute) until breathing resumes.

- ► If adequate breathing resumes and head or neck trauma is not suspected, place the child in the recovery position.
- Begin chest compressions if there is no pulse or if the heart rate is less than 60 beats/min with signs of poor perfusion.

Chest Compressions—Infant

- Imagine a line between the nipples. Place the flat part of your middle and ring fingers about one finger width below this imaginary line.
- Press down on the sternum and deliver 30 compressions at a rate of about 100 per minute. Apply firm pressure, depressing the sternum about $1/3$ to $1/2$ the depth of the chest. Do not apply pressure over the bottom tip of the sternum (xiphoid process) or over the upper abdomen.
- After 30 compressions, open the airway and give two breaths.
- Continue compressions and breaths in a ratio of 30 to 2 until the infant shows obvious signs of life, advanced life support personnel arrive and take over, you are too exhausted to continue, or a physician instructs you to stop.

Chest Compression—Child

- Find the lower half of the sternum (center of the chest between the nipples) and place the heel of one hand there. If the child is large or more than 8 years of age, use two hands to compress the chest and ensure an adequate depth of compression (i.e., the technique used for adults).

- Position yourself directly over the child's chest. With your arms straight and your elbows locked, press down on the sternum and deliver 30 compressions at a rate of about 100 per minute. Apply firm pressure, depressing the sternum $1/3$ to $1/2$ the depth of the chest. Do not apply pressure over the bottom tip of the sternum or over the upper abdomen.
- After 30 compressions, open the airway and give two breaths.
- Continue compressions and breaths in a ratio of 30 to 2 until the victim shows obvious signs of life, advanced life support personnel arrive and take over, you are too exhausted to continue, or a physician instructs you to stop.
- If an automated external defibrillator (AED) is available, attach the device and follow the machine's instructions/prompts.

Medications Used for CPR

	POSITIVE INOTROPE	POSITIVE CHRONOTROPE	DIRECT PRESSOR	VASODILATOR
Dopamine	++	+	±	++*
Dobutamine	++	±	-	+
Epinephrine	+++	+++	+++	-
Isoproterenol	+++	+++	-	+++
Norepinephrine	+++	+++	+++	-

*Primarily splanchnic and renal in low doses (3 to 5 mcg/kg/min)

From Krug SE: The acutely ill or injured child. In Behrman RE, Kliegman RM, editors: Nelson essentials of pediatrics, ed 4, Philadelphia, 2002, Saunders.

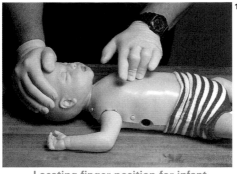

Locating finger position for infant
chest compression

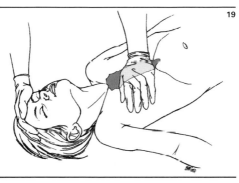

Locating hand position for child
chest compression

Infant and Child CPR—2 Rescuers

EMS professionals usually work in teams of
at least two and arrive simultaneously on the
scene of an emergency. Typically, one rescuer establishes unresponsiveness, assesses
and opens the airway, and proceeds with the

indicated care. The other rescuer quickly prepares equipment such as suction, oxygen, and ventilation devices. The second rescuer (or third rescuer when available) also performs external chest compressions when indicated. Whenever two rescuers are present and are not responding EMS professionals, one rescuer should provide CPR while the second rescuer activates EMS.[4]

CPR PERFORMED BY TWO (OR MORE) RESCUERS

- Establish unresponsiveness.

Rescuer 1

- ▶ Open the airway (head tilt—chin lift or jaw thrust without head tilt maneuver).
- ▶ Look, listen, and feel for breathing.
- ▶ Give 2 breaths (1 second each) if breathing is absent or inadequate. Be sure the chest rises with each breath and allow for exhalation between breaths.
- ▶ Check for a pulse. Assess the brachial or femoral pulse in infants. Assess the carotid pulse in a child.
- ▶ If a pulse is present but the infant or child is not breathing, give rescue breaths at a rate of 1 breath every 3 to 5 seconds (12 to 20/minute) until breathing resumes.

Rescuer 2

- ▶ If no pulse is present or if the heart rate is less than 60 beats/min with signs of poor perfusion, perform chest compressions.
  - ○ For an infant, encircle the chest with both hands and compress the sternum between your opposing thumbs (or use the finger position previously described for single-rescuer infant

CPR) at a rate of about 100 per minute.
Apply firm pressure, depressing the
sternum about $1/2$ to 1 inch. Your
thumbs should be positioned about

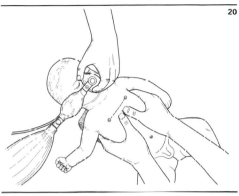

20

Two-rescuer infant CPR, two thumb–
encircling hands technique

one finger width below the nipple line.
○ For a child, use the same technique
  used for single-rescuer child CPR at a
  rate of about 100 per minute. Apply
  firm pressure, depressing the sternum
  $1/3$ to $1/2$ the depth of the chest.
○ Deliver 15 chest compressions, pausing for a breath delivered by rescuer 1
  Once an advanced airway is in place,
  do not pause compressions for a
  breath. Ventilate at a rate of 8 to
  10/minute.
• Rescuer #1 should provide oxygen by
  means of a pediatric bag-valve-mask
  device or CPR mask.

INDICATIONS

- Maintaining hydration
- Restoring fluid and electrolyte balance
- Providing fluids for resuscitation
- Administration of medications, volume expanders, blood and blood components, maintenance solutions
- Obtaining venous blood specimens for laboratory analysis

GENERAL PRINCIPLES

- In the management of cardiopulmonary arrest and decompensated shock, the preferred vascular access site is the largest, most readily accessible vein.
  - If no IV is in place at the onset of a cardiac arrest, attempt to establish vascular access at a site that will not interrupt resuscitation efforts.
  - If a central line is in place when an arrest occurs, it should be used for drug administration during the resuscitation effort.
- The preferred IV solutions in cardiac arrest are normal saline or lactated Ringer's solution. Large volumes of dextrose-containing solutions should not be infused because hyperglycemia may induce osmotic diuresis, produce or aggravate hyperkalemia, and worsen ischemic brain injury.

- Medications administered via a peripheral vein during CPR should be followed with a saline flush of 5 to 10 mL to facilitate delivery of the medication to the central circulation.

INTRAOSSEOUS (IO) INFUSION

Intraosseous infusion (IOI) is the process of infusing medications, fluids, and blood products into the bone marrow cavity. Because the marrow cavity is continuous with the venous circulation, fluids and medications administered by the IO route are subsequently delivered to the venous circulation.

In the presence of cardiac arrest or decompensated shock, an intraosseous infusion should be established in any patient when IV access cannot be achieved rapidly. IOI is a temporary means of vascular access. The duration of the infusion should be limited to a few hours. Venous access is often easier to obtain after initial fluid and medication resuscitation via the intraosseous route.

Indications

- Cardiopulmonary arrest or decompensated shock in which vascular access is essential and venous access is not readily achieved
- Multisystem trauma with associated shock and/or severe hypovolemia
- Unresponsive patient in need of immediate medications or fluid resuscitation (e.g., burns, sepsis, near-drowning, anaphylaxis, status epilepticus)
- Presence of burns or a traumatic injury preventing access to the venous system at other sites

Advantages

- Skill is easily mastered, even if done infrequently; healthcare professionals experienced in the technique can often establish IO access in 60 seconds or less
- Preferred access sites are distant from major sites of activity during resuscitation efforts
- Low incidence of complications
- Medications and fluids administered IV can be administered IO
- Absorption of medications administered via the IO route is more rapid than medications administered via the subcutaneous or rectal routes
- Blood sampling for lab studies is possible
- Venous access is often easier to obtain after initial fluid resuscitation via the intraosseous route

Disadvantages

- Short term intervention until venous access can be obtained
- Extremely painful for responsive patients

Contraindications

- Femoral fracture on the ipsilateral side
- Osteopetrosis (high fracture potential)
- Osteogenesis imperfecta (high fracture potential)
- Fracture at or above the insertion site
- Severe burn overlying the insertion site (unless this is the only available site)
- Infection at insertion site (unless this is the only available site)
- Use of the same bone in which an unsuccessful IO attempt was previously made

AUTOMATED EXTERNAL DEFIBRILLATION

An automated external defibrillator (AED) is an external defibrillator with a computerized cardiac rhythm analysis system. The patient's cardiac rhythm is analyzed by a microprocessor in the defibrillator that uses an algorithm to distinguish rhythms that should be shocked from those that do not require defibrillation. Some AEDs require the operator to press an "analyze" control to initiate rhythm analysis, whereas others automatically begin analyzing the patient's cardiac rhythm when the electrode pads are attached to the patient's chest.

Standard AEDs should be used for patients that are apneic, pulseless, and ≥8 years of age (approximately >25 kg body weight). Several AED manufacturers have designed pediatric pad/cable systems for use with AEDs designed for use in adults to reduce the energy delivered to patients less than 8 years of age. If a child between the ages of 1 and 8 experiences a cardiac arrest and an AED with a pediatric pad/cable system is not available, use a standard AED.

Medical science now supports early defibrillation for children with a pediatric-ready AED. However, there is currently insufficient evidence to support a recommendation for or against the use of AEDs in children less than 1 year of age.[5] Always follow the AED manufacturer's guidelines for the application, use, and maintenance of the AED.[6]

AED Operation

- Use personal protective equipment.
- Assess responsiveness.
- Open the airway and check for breathing. If the patient is not breathing, deliver two slow breaths.
- Assess for the presence of a pulse. If the patient is pulseless, begin chest compressions and attach the AED.
- Turn on the power to the AED. Depending on the brand of AED, this is accomplished by either pressing the "on" button or lifting up the monitor screen or lid.
  - ▶ Open the package containing the self-adhesive monitoring/defibrillation pads. Connect the pads to the AED cables (if not preconnected), and then apply the pads to the patient's torso in the locations specified by the AED manufacturer. Momentarily stop CPR to allow placement of the pads.
  - ▶ Some models require connection of the AED cable to the AED before use.
- Analyze the ECG rhythm.
  - ▶ AEDs take multiple "looks" at the patient's rhythm, each lasting a few seconds. If several "looks" confirm the presence of a shockable rhythm, the AED will signal that a shock is indicated.
  - ▶ Artifact due to motion or 60-cycle interference can simulate VF and interfere with accurate rhythm analysis. While the AED is analyzing the patient's cardiac rhythm, all movement (including chest compressions, artificial ventilations, and the movement associated with patient transport) must cease.

- Clear the area surrounding the patient. Be sure to look around you.
  - ▸ Ensure that everyone is clear of the patient, bed, and any equipment connected to the patient.
  - ▸ Ensure that oxygen is not flowing over the patient's torso (increases risk of spark/fire).
- If the area is clear, press the shock control to deliver the shock. After delivering the shock, immediately resume CPR, starting with chest compressions.

Electrical Therapy

INTERVENTION	DYSRHYTHMIA	RECOMMENDED ENERGY LEVELS
Defibrillation	• Pulseless VT/VF	• 2 J/kg, 4 J/kg, 4 J/kg (or equivalent biphasic energy)
Synchronized cardioversion	• Supraventricular tachycardia (SVT) • Atrial flutter with a rapid ventricular response • VT with a pulse	• 0.5 to 1 J/kg, 2 J/kg (or equivalent biphasic energy)
Transcutaneous pacing	• Severe bradycardia (e.g., complete AV block)	• Set initial rate at 100 pulses/min • Increase output (mA) until pacer spikes are visible before each QRS complex. Verify capture. • Final mA setting should be slightly above where capture is obtained to help prevent loss of capture.

FLUIDS & MEDICATIONS

MEDICATION ADMINISTRATION

- When possible, use a length-based resuscitation tape to determine the correct dosage for medication administration or fluid resuscitation in children.

- Check each medication at least three times before administering it.

  ► Check the medication when removing it from its storage container (i.e., drug box, code cart).

  ► Check the medication again when preparing it for administration.

  ► Check it once more at the patient's side before administering it.

- Question any medication dosage that is outside the normal range.

- Using age-appropriate language, explain to the child (and parents) why a medication is necessary.

- Children should always be praised for cooperating in taking their medications.

- If the child is uncooperative, restrain the child as necessary.

Medication errors are common and preventable. Make it a habit to have a co-worker double-check your medication and dosage before administering it to an infant or child. This is particularly important for controlled substances (e.g., narcotics, sedatives), antiarrhythmics, heparin, insulin, and medications used during resuscitation.

■ PAIN MANAGEMENT & SEDATION ■

PAIN TERMINOLOGY

The following list of terms and definitions related to pain is from the International Association for the Study of Pain.[7]

- Pain: an unpleasant sensory and emotional experience associated with actual or potential tissue damage, or described in terms of such damage. The inability to communicate verbally does not negate the possibility that an individual is experiencing pain and is in need of appropriate pain-relieving treatment

- Pain threshold: the least experience of pain that a subject can recognize

- Pain tolerance level: the greatest level of pain that a subject is prepared to tolerate

- Analgesia: absence of pain in response to stimulation that would normally be painful[1]

Because no individual can feel another's pain, "Pain is whatever the experiencing person says it is, existing whenever s/he says it does."[8] The patient, not the healthcare professional, is the authority regarding his or her pain.

Sympathetic (Adrenergic) Receptors

	ALPHA-1	ALPHA-2	BETA-1	BETA-2	DOPAMINERGIC
Location	Vascular smooth muscle	Skeletal blood vessels	Myocardium	Predominantly in bronchiolar and arterial smooth muscle	Coronary arteries, renal, mesenteric, and visceral blood vessels
Effects of stimulation	Vasoconstriction; peripheral vascular resistance	Inhibits norepinephrine release	Heart rate Myocardial contractility Oxygen consumption	Relaxation of bronchial smooth muscle arteriolar dilation	Dilation

119

Tracheal Medication Administration

Advantages	• Permits delivery of lipid-soluble medications into the pulmonary alveoli and systemic circulation via lung capillaries
Disadvantages	• Limited number of medications can be administered via this route • Medication absorption may be negatively affected by presence of blood, emesis, or secretions in trachea or tracheal tube • No fluid resuscitation possible via this medication route
Examples	• Remember "NAVEL:" Naloxone, Atropine, Vasopressin, Epinephrine, Lidocaine
Notes	• Use the tracheal route for medication administration during resuscitation efforts if a tracheal tube is in place but IV or IO access is not available. • When administering medications by means of a tracheal tube, temporarily stop chest compressions and instill the medication down the tracheal tube. Follow the drug with a flush of 5 mL of normal saline and 5 positive-pressure ventilations, and then resume CPR. • Some medications may cause false end-tidal CO_2 detector readings when administered via the tracheal route.[12]

Volume Expansion: Summary

Crystalloid solutions

Description	Isotonic solutions that provide transient expansion of the intravascular volume
Examples	Normal saline: contains sodium chloride in water Ringer's lactate: contains sodium chloride, potassium chloride, calcium chloride, and sodium lactate in water
Advantages	Inexpensive, readily available, free from allergic reactions
Disadvantages	Effectively expand the interstitial space and correct sodium deficits but do not effectively expand the intravascular volume because approximately three fourths of the infused crystalloid solution leaves the vascular space in about 1 hour

Colloid solutions

Description	Contain molecules (typically proteins) that are too large to pass out of the capillary membranes. As a result, they remain in the vascular compartment and draw fluid from the interstitial and intracellular compartments into the vascular compartment to expand the intravascular volume.
Examples	5% albumin, fresh frozen plasma; synthetic colloids include hetastarch and Dextran
Advantages	More efficient than crystalloid solutions in rapidly expanding the intravascular compartment; remain in the intravascular space for hours.
Disadvantages	Expensive, short shelf-life, potential for adverse reactions; can produce dramatic fluid shifts

Blood

Indications	Correction of a deficiency or functional defect of a blood component that has caused a clinically significant problem severe acute hemorrhage
Notes	Red blood cells (RBCs) are the most frequently transfused blood component, given to increase the oxygen-carrying capacity of the blood and to maintain satisfactory tissue oxygenation. If blood is administered, it should be warmed before transfusion otherwise, rapid administration may result in significant hypothermia.

Intramuscular Injection Sites in Children

SITE	AGE	NEEDLE	CONSIDERATIONS
Vastus lateralis	Preferred site for infants and children <3 years, but may be used in all ages	Use 22-25 gauge, ⅝ inch to 1 inch needle inserted at a 90-degree angle to site	• No nearby major nerves or vessels • Large, easily accessible muscle • Can inject up to 0.5 mL of fluid in infant, 2 mL in child
Ventrogluteal	Consider for children >3 years of age	Use 22-25 gauge ½ inch to 1 inch needle inserted almost perpendicular to site but angled slightly (10 to 15 degrees) toward iliac crest	• No nearby major nerves or vessels • Prominent bony landmarks • Thin layer of Subq tissue • Can inject up to 0.5 mL of fluid in infant, 2 mL in child • Healthcare professional is often unfamiliar with site
Dorsogluteal	Contraindicated for children <3 years of age and nonambulatory patients	Use 20-25 gauge ½ inch to 1½ inch needle inserted perpendicular to surface on which the child is lying when prone	• Risk of damage to sciatic nerve • Depth of overlying Subq tissue varies • Well-developed muscle in older child can tolerate fluid volume of up to 2 mL
Deltoid	Toddler, preschooler, older child, adolescent	Use 22-25 gauge ½ inch to 1 inch needle inserted at a 90-degree angle to site	• Small muscle mass can tolerate only small fluid volume (0.5 to 1 mL) • Faster absorption than gluteal sites • Easily accessible • Possible damage to radial and axillary nerves

PAIN ASSESSMENT IN INFANTS AND CHILDREN

Methods for assessing pain in the pediatric patient vary according to the age of the child. One approach to pain assessment is QUESTT[9]:

Question the child

Use pain rating scales

Evaluate behavior and physiologic changes

Secure parents' involvement

Take cause of pain into account

Take action

- Use an age-appropriate pain rating scale.
  - ► Many assessment tools are available. All providers caring for the child should use the same scale consistently.
  - ► Assessment tools include, but are not limited to:
- The Children's Hospital of Eastern Ontario Pain Scale (CHEOPS) was one of the earliest tools developed to assess pain behaviors in young children. CHEOPS incorporates six categories of behavior that are scored individually (range of 0 to 2 or 1 to 3) and then totaled for a pain score ranging from 4 to 13.
- The Wong-Baker FACES Pain Rating Scale combines three scales into one: facial expressions, numbers, and words. The scale consists of 6 cartoon faces ranging from a smiling face depicting "no hurt" to a tearful, sad face illustrating "worst hurt." The FACES Scale is best used for children three years or older.

- The Oucher Scale consists of a vertical numerical scale (10 to 100) for children who can count to 100 and a vertical photographic scale of a child with expressions of "no hurt" to "worst hurt."
- The Color Scale. Using markers or crayons, the child is asked to select a color that is like their "worst or most hurt," a color that is like "a little less hurt," a color for "even less hurt" and finally, a color for "no hurt." A numeric value is then placed on each color.

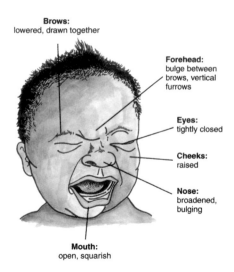

Brows: lowered, drawn together

Forehead: bulge between brows, vertical furrows

Eyes: tightly closed

Cheeks: raised

Nose: broadened, bulging

Mouth: open, squarish

From Hockenberry M, Wilson D, Winkelstein M, Kline N; Wong's Nursing Care of Infants and Children, 7e. St. Louis, 2002, Mosby.

PEDIATRIC PAIN ASSESSMENT[21]

Wong-Baker FACES Pain Rating Scale

Brief word instructions: Point to each face using the words to describe the pain intensity. Ask the child to choose face that best describes his or her pain and record the appropriate number.

(From Hockenberry MJ: Wong's nursing care of infants and children, ed 7, St Louis, 2003. Mosby. Reprinted by permission.)

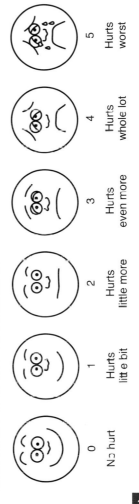

0	1	2	3	4	5
No hurt	Hurts little bit	Hurts little more	Hurts even more	Hurts whole lot	Hurts worst

Fallacies and Facts about Children and Pain

FALLACY	FACT
Infants do not feel pain.	Infants demonstrate behavioral (especially facial), and physiologic (including hormonal), indicators of pain. Fetuses have the neural mechanisms to transmit noxious stimuli by 20 weeks of gestation.
Children tolerate pain better than adults do.	A child's tolerance for pain increases with age. Younger children tend to rate procedure-related pain higher than older children do.
Children cannot tell you where they hurt.	By 4 years of age, children can accurately point to the body area or mark the painful site on a drawing. Children as young as 3 years old can use pain scales, such as FACES.
Children always tell the truth about pain.	Children may not admit having pain to avoid an injection. Because of constant pain, they may not realize how much they are hurting. Children may believe that others know how they are feeling and not ask for analgesia.
Children become accustomed to pain or painful procedures.	Children often demonstrate increased behavioral signs of discomfort with repeated painful procedures.
Behavioral manifestations reflect pain intensity.	A child's developmental level, coping abilities, and temperament (e.g., activity level and intensity of reaction to pain) influence pain behavior. Children with more active, resisting behaviors may rate pain lower than children with passive, accepting behaviors.
Narcotics are more dangerous for children than they are for adults.	Narcotics (opioids) are no more dangerous for children than they are for adults. Addiction to opioids used to treat pain is extremely rare in children. Reports of respiratory depression in children are also uncommon. By 3 to 6 months of age, healthy infants can metabolize opioids like other children.

Adapted from Hockenberry MJ, Wilson D, Winkelstein ML, Kline KE: Wong's nursing care of infants and children, ed 7, St. Louis, 2003, Mosby, p 1049.

Nonpharmacologic Methods of Pain Management

AGE	NONPHARMACOLOGIC TECHNIQUE
• Infant (1 to 12 months)	• Allow caregiver to remain with the child • Promote relaxation with rocking, holding, light massage • Allow the infant to suck on a pacifier • Distract infant with finger puppets, a rattle, plastic keys, music box, singing • Cover injuries or deformities
• Toddler (1 to 3 years)	• Allow caregiver to remain with the child • Promote relaxation with rocking, holding, light massage • Distract child with singing, listening to music, making funny faces, playing with a favorite toy, finger puppets, telling a story, using pop-up books or books with sound effects • Cover injuries or deformities
• Preschooler (4 to 5 years)	• Allow caregiver to remain with the child • Promote relaxation with rocking, holding, light massage • Distract child with singing, listening to music, making funny faces, playing with a favorite toy, finger puppets, telling a story, using pop-up books with sound effects • Deep breathing exercises • Cover injuries or deformities
• School-age (6 to 12 years)	• Allow caregiver to remain with the child • Have child visualize being in a "safe" or "beautiful" place • Deep breathing exercises • Cover injuries or deformities • Progressive muscle relaxation • Distract child with humor, telling stories, watching cartoons, playing games, or listening to familiar music on a tape or CD
• Adolescent (13 to 18 years)	• Allow caregiver to remain with the child, if child and caregiver desire • Have child visualize being in a tranquil place • Deep breathing exercises, rhythmic breathing • Progressive muscle relaxation • Distract child with humor, watching a favorite movie, playing games, or listening to familiar music on a tape or CD • Cover injuries or deformities

Levels of Sedation/Analgesia

LEVEL	DESCRIPTION	COMMENTS
Minimal	• Anxiety is reduced; cognitive function and coordination may be impaired • Protective reflexes present • Able to maintain patent airway independently and continuously • Able to respond appropriately to verbal command (e.g., "Open your eyes.") • Ventilatory and cardiovascular functions intact	• Equivalent to anxiolysis • Examples of minimal sedation/analgesia include peripheral nerve blocks; local or topical anesthesia; or a single, oral sedative or analgesic medication administered in doses appropriate for the unsupervised treatment of insomnia, anxiety, or pain
Moderate	• Level of consciousness minimally depressed • Protective reflexes present; able to maintain patent airway independently and continuously • Spontaneous ventilation is adequate • Able to respond purposefully to verbal command (e.g., "Open your eyes."), either alone or accompanied by light tactile stimulation; reflex withdrawal from a painful stimulus is NOT considered a purposeful response • Cardiovascular function is usually maintained	• Equivalent to conscious sedation • Risk of potential loss of protective reflexes exists • May be accompanied by loss of protective reflexes and ventilatory drive

Deep	• Drug-induced state of depressed consciousness	• Assistance may be required to maintain a patent airway
	• Cannot be easily aroused but responds purposefully after repeated or painful stimulation; reflex withdrawal from a painful stimulus is NOT considered a purposeful response	• Positive pressure ventilation may be required
	• Ability to maintain ventilatory function independently may be impaired	
	• Spontaneous ventilation may be inadequate	
	• Cardiovascular function is usually maintained	
General anesthesia	• Drug-induced state of unconsciousness	• Assistance often required to maintain a patent airway
	• Unable to maintain patent airway independently	• Positive pressure ventilation may be required
	• Not arousable, even by painful stimulation	
	• Ability to maintain ventilatory function independently is often impaired	
	• Cardiovascular function may be impaired	

Fasting Recommendations Before Elective Procedures

INGESTED MATERIAL	MINIMUM FASTING PERIOD
Clear liquids Examples: water, fruit juices without pulp, carbonated beverages, clear tea, black coffee	2 hours
Breast milk	4 hours
Infant formula	6 hours
Nonhuman milk Since nonhuman milk is similar to solids in gastric emptying time, the amount ingested must be considered in determining an appropriate fasting period.	6 hours
Light meal A light meal typically consists of toast and clear liquids. Meals that include fried or fatty foods or meat may prolong gastric emptying time. Both the amount and type of foods ingested must be considered in determining an appropriate fasting period.	6 hours

Developed by the American Society of Anesthesiologists. These recommendations apply to healthy patients who are undergoing elective procedures. Following these recommendations does not guarantee that complete gastric emptying has occurred.

Medications Used for Sedation/Analgesia

	Sedation	Amnesia	Analgesia
BARBITURATES	☺ ☺ ☺		

Methohexital (Brevital)
- Administered rectally
- Faster onset of action and recovery time than thiopental, and twice as potent
- May precipitate seizures
- Use with extreme caution in patients in status asthmaticus
- Onset 5-15 minutes; duration 30-90 minutes

Pentobarbital (Nembutal)
- Can increase pain perception; not useful as a sedative during painful procedures
- Onset IV 1-5 minutes, duration 15-60 minutes
- Onset IM 5-15 minutes, duration 2-4 hours
- Onset PO 15-60 minutes, duration 2-4 hours

Thiopental (Pentothal)
- Administered rectally
- Onset 5-15 minutes; duration 60-90 minutes

	Sedation	Amnesia	Analgesia
BENZODIAZEPINES	☺ ☺ ☺	☺ ☺ ☺	

Diazepam (Valium)
- Sedative effects reversible with flumazenil
- Fat soluble
- Respiratory depressant effects are potentiated when administered in conjunction with opioids
- Slow administration decreases incidence of respiratory side effects and venous irritation
- Onset IV 2-3 minutes, duration 30-90 minutes; half-life about 30 hours
- Onset per rectum 5-15 minutes, duration 2-4 hours

Lorazepam (Ativan)
- Sedative effects reversible with flumazenil
- Respiratory depressant effects are potentiated when administered in conjunction with opioids
- IV administration can cause venous irritation
- Onset IV 3-5 minutes, duration 2-6 hours
- Onset IM 10-20 minutes, duration 2-6 hours
- Onset PO 60 minutes, duration 2-6 hours

continued

Midazolam (Versed)

- Sedative effects reversible with flumazenil
- Water soluble
- 2-4 times more potent than diazepam and provides deeper sedation and more amnesia than diazepam
- Respiratory depressant effects are potentiated when administered in conjunction with opioids; respiratory depression is related to dosage given and rate of administration: the faster the drug is given, the more likely apnea will result
- Compatible with many IV solutions and other medications; IV administration does not result in venous irritation
- Onset IV 1-2 minutes, duration 30-60 minutes; onset IM 5-15 minutes, duration 30-60 minutes; onset per rectum 5-10 minutes, duration 30-60 minutes; onset PO 10 minutes, duration 1-2 hours

	Sedation	Amnesia	Analgesia
OPIOIDS (NARCOTICS)	☺ ☺		☺ ☺ ☺

Fentanyl (Sublimaze)

- Respiratory depression reversible with naloxone
- Synthetic opioid used for pain or anxiety associated with short procedures
- 50-100 times more powerful than morphine; recheck dosage carefully before administering
- Causes minimal or no release of histamine
- Infants <3 months of age may be more sensitive to respiratory depressant effects
- Respiratory depressant effects are potentiated when administered in conjunction with benzodiazepines
- Chest wall rigidity may occur with large doses given rapidly
- Onset IV 2 minutes; duration IV 20-60 minutes; half-life about 20 minutes

Morphine

- Respiratory depression reversible with naloxone
- Used as a standard of comparison for all opioids
- Can stimulate histamine release
- Respiratory depressant effects are potentiated when administered in conjunction with benzodiazepines
- Hypovolemia makes the occurrence of hemodynamic side effects more common
- Onset IV 5-10 minutes; duration IV 2-4 hours

OTHER AGENTS	Sedation	Amnesia	Analgesia
Chloral hydrate	☺ ☺		

- Sedative/hypnotic used for pediatric sedation for more than 100 years
- Used primarily for sedation for painless diagnostic procedures (e.g., MRI scan)
- Has CNS, respiratory, and cardiovascular depressant effects
- Increased risk of respiratory depression when administered concurrently with opioids or benzodiazepines
- Paradoxical agitation may occur; more likely in children with underlying developmental delays or neurologic disorders
- Onset PO or per rectum 15-30 minutes, duration 2-3 hours

	Sedation	Amnesia	Analgesia
Ketamine (Ketalar)	☺ ☺ ☺	☺	☺ ☺ ☺

- Used for sedation during painful procedures
- Derivative of phencyclidine
- Child may appear awake with eyes open despite deep sedation
- May cause hypertension, hypotension, emergence reactions, tachycardia, laryngospasm, respiratory depression, and stimulation of salivary secretions
- Onset IV 1-2 minutes, duration 15-60 minutes; onset IM 3-10 minutes, duration 15-60 minutes

	Sedation	Amnesia	Analgesia
Ketorolac (Toradol)			☺ ☺ ☺

- Nonsteroidal anti-inflammatory drug (NSAID) used for moderate to severe pain
- IV route of administration in children is not yet recommended by the manufacturer, although it is well supported in the literature and in clinical practice
- Onset IV 10-15 minutes, duration 3-6 hours

	Sedation	Amnesia	Analgesia
Propofol (Diprivan)	☺ ☺ ☺	☺	

- Used for sedation during procedures not associated with pain
- Potent vasodilator, cardiac depressant, and respiratory depressant
- Short duration of action necessitates administration by continuous IV infusion
- Insoluble in water
- Onset IV 1-2 minutes, duration 3-5 minutes

Pharmacologic Antagonists (Reversal Agents)

Agent	Remarks
Naloxone (opioid antagonist)	• Effective for all opioids (narcotics) • Effects of narcotics are usually longer than those of naloxone; therefore respiratory depression may return when naloxone has worn off. Monitor the patient closely and observe continuously for resedation for at least 2 hours after the last dose of naloxone.
Flumazenil (benzodiazepine antagonist)	• Effective for all benzodiazepines • Observe continuously for resedation for at least 2 hours after the last dose of flumazenil. • Administer as a series of small injections (not as a single bolus injection) to control the reversal of sedation to the approximate endpoint desired and minimize the possibility of adverse effects. • Safety and efficacy in reversal of moderate sedation/analgesia in pediatric patients below 1 year of age has not been established.

Common Medications Used in Pediatric Emergency Care

MEDICATION	INDICATION(S)
Adenosine (Adenocard)	• Supraventricular tachycardia (SVT)
Albuterol (Proventil, Ventolin)	• Bronchospasm, status asthmaticus
Amiodarone (Cordarone)	• Pulseless VT/VF • Perfusing tachycardias, particularly ectopic atrial tachycardia, junctional ectopic tachycardia, and ventricular tachycardia
Atropine sulfate	• Symptomatic bradycardia • Anticholinesterase poisoning • To reduce secretions during rapid-sequence intubation (RSI) or block reflex bradycardia induced by succinylcholine and laryngoscopy during RSI
Calcium	• Ionized hypocalcemia • Hyperkalemia • Hypermagnesemia • Calcium channel blocker toxicity
Charcoal, activated	• Acute ingestion of selected toxic substances
Chloral hydrate	• Sedation
Dexamethasone (Decadron)	• Moderate to severe croup
Diazepam (Valium)	• Status epilepticus • Extreme anxiety or agitation
Digoxin (Lanoxin)	• Heart failure due to poor left ventricular contractility
Diphenhydramine (Benadryl)	• Anaphylaxis • Dystonic reactions
Dobutamine (Dobutrex) infusion	• Impaired cardiac contractility • Cardiogenic shock
Dopamine (Intropin, Dopastat) infusion	• Persistent hypotension or shock after volume resuscitation and stable cardiac rhythm • Inadequate cardiac output • Cardiogenic shock, septic shock

continued

Common Medications Used in Pediatric Emergency Care (continued)

MEDICATION	INDICATION(S)
Epinephrine for bradycardia	• Symptomatic bradycardia unresponsive to oxygenation and ventilation
Epinephrine for bronchospasm	• Asthma/reactive airway disease • Anaphylaxis
Epinephrine for asystolic or pulseless arrest	• Pulseless ventricular tachycardia • Ventricular fibrillation • Asystole • Pulseless electrical activity
Epinephrine infusion	• Continued shock after volume resuscitation
Etomidate (Amidate)	• Sedative used in rapid sequence intubation
Fentanyl (Sublimaze)	• Pain • Sedative used in (RSI)
Flumazenil (Romazicon)	• Benzodiazepine intoxication
Furosemide (Lasix)	• Congestive heart failure • Fluid overload
Glucose	• Hypoglycemia
Glycopyrrolate (Robinul)	• Adjunctive medication that may be used during RSI
Ipratropium bromide (Atrovent)	• May be beneficial for moderate to severe exacerbations of asthma
Ketamine (Ketalar)	• Sedation/analgesia • Adjunct to rapid sequence intubation
Ketorolac (Toradol)	• Moderate to severe pain
Lidocaine	• Ventricular tachycardia, ventricular fibrillation • Adjunctive agent in rapid sequence intubation
Lidocaine infusion	• Ventricular tachycardia, ventricular fibrillation
Lorazepam (Ativan)	• Status epilepticus • Adjunct for intubation
Magnesium sulfate	• Torsade de pointes (TDP) • Severe asthma

MEDICATION	INDICATION(S)
Methohexital (Brevital)	• Sedation
Methylprednisolone (Solu-Medrol)	• Reactive airway disease • Anaphylaxis • Croup
Midazolam (Versed)	• Sedative used in RSI • Sedation/anxiolysis
Morphine sulfate	• Pain • "Tet spell"
Naloxone (Narcan)	• Coma of unknown etiology to rule out (or reverse) opioid-induced coma • Opiate induced respiratory depression
Nitrous oxide	• Moderate to severe pain
Nitroprusside (Nipride) infusion	• Immediate reduction of blood pressure in a hypertensive emergency or hypertensive urgency
Norepinephrine (Levophed) infusion	• Inadequate cardiac output • Septic shock, neurogenic shock, anaphylaxis, drug overdose with significant alpha-adrenergic blocking effects (e.g., tricyclic antidepressants)
Oxygen	• All arrest situations • Hypoxemia and/or respiratory distress • Carbon monoxide poisoning • Shock
Pancuronium (Pavulon)	• Nondepolarizing agent used during RSI
Pentobarbital (Pronestyl)	• Sedation
Procainamide (Pronestyl)	• Ventricular tachycardia with a pulse
Propofol (Diprivan)	• Sedation • Sedative/hypnotic used in rapid sequence intubation (RSI)
Prostaglandin E$_1$ Infusion	• Possible ductal-dependent cardiac malformation in a neonate
Rocuronium (Zemuron)	• Nondepolarizing agent used during RSI

continued

Common Medications Used in Pediatric Emergency Care (continued)

MEDICATION	INDICATION(S)
Sodium bicarbonate	• Severe metabolic acidosis • Tricyclic antidepressant overdose • Hyperkalemia
Succinylcholine (Anectine)	• Depolarizing agent used during RSI
Thiopental (Pentothal)	• Sedative used in RSI • Sedation
Vecuronium (Norcuron)	• Nondepolarizing agent used during RSI
Verapamil (Isoptin, Calan)	• Supraventricular tachycardia

Common Childhood Injuries

AGE	COMMON CHILDHOOD INJURIES
Infant	Child abuse, burns, falls, drowning
Toddler	Burns, drowning, falls, poisonings
School-age	Pedestrian injuries, bicycle-related injuries (the most serious usually involve motor vehicles), motor vehicle occupant injuries, burns, drowning
Adolescent	Motor vehicle occupant trauma, drowning, burns, intentional trauma, work-related injuries

THORACIC INJURIES

Immediately life-threatening injuries that must be identified and managed in the primary survey include:

- Airway obstruction
- Open pneumothorax
- Tension pneumothorax
- Massive hemothorax
- Flail chest
- Cardiac tamponade

SPINAL TRAUMA

SPINAL STABILIZATION INDICATIONS

- Mechanisms of injury involving blunt or penetrating trauma directly to the spine or forces applied to the spine involving flexion, extension, or rotation of the head and neck (e.g., sports injuries, falls from heights)

- A mechanism of injury that may have resulted in rapid, forceful head movement
- Consider in any child with an altered mental status and no history available, found in setting of possible trauma, or near drowning with history or probability of diving
- Neurologic deficit in the arms or legs
- Significant helmet damage
- Local tenderness or deformity in the cervical, thoracic, or lumbar region

RADIOGRAPHIC EVALUATION OF THE CERVICAL SPINE[10]

Pre-Verbal or Pre-Cooperative Child at Risk of Cervical Spine Injury (CSI)

- High Risk
  - ▶ Fall in which the body weight lands on the head
  - ▶ Head-on motor vehicle crash with child in a forward-facing seat
  - ▶ Abnormal posture of the head and neck
  - ▶ Anomaly of the face, head, or neck
  - ▶ Any suspicion of nonaccidental trauma
  - ▶ Evidence of intracranial injury or significant facial trauma
  - ▶ High speed, rear-end impact with an infant in a rear-facing seat
  - ▶ Risky mechanism with distracting pain
  - ▶ Neck tenderness
  - ▶ Neurologic deficit
  - ▶ Fall while in an infant walker

- Low Risk
  - ▶ Head-on motor vehicle crash with child in a rear-facing seat
  - ▶ Short fall in which impact is evenly dis-

tributed between trunk and head
- ► Unwitnessed short fall with no scalp hematoma or soft-tissue injury
- ► Lateral impact motor vehicle crash with the child in appropriate restraint and no evidence of intracranial injury or concussion

Verbal and Cooperative Child at Risk for Cervical Spine Injury

- Neck tenderness
- Neurologic abnormality
- Distracting pain with adequate mechanism
- Altered mental status
- High-energy impact involving a child younger than 8 years of age

TRAUMA

PEDIATRIC TRAUMA SCORE

The pediatric trauma score (PTS) is a scoring tool used to evaluate the severity of injury in the pediatric patient and assist in pediatric triage decisions. The PTS consists of six parameters that are evaluated during the initial assessment of an injured child. Each parameter is assessed and given a numeric score based on three variables: +2 (no injury or non-life threatening), +1 (minor injury or potentially life threatening), or -1 (life threatening). The scores are then added together. Children with a PTS of <8 should be treated in a designated trauma center.

Pediatric Trauma Score[15]

CLINICAL CATEGORY	SCORE		
	2	1	-1
Size	Child/adolescent >20 kg (44 lbs.)	Toddler 10-20 kg (22 to 44 lbs.)	Infant <10 kg (22 lbs.)
Airway	Patent; no assistance required	Maintainable by patient but observation needed to ensure adequate airway (e.g., positioning, suctioning)	Unmaintainable airway devices needed to maintain airway (e.g., oral airway, tracheal tube, cricothyroidotomy)
Mental status (AVPU)	Awake; no loss of consciousness	Obtunded; responds to verbal or painful stimulus; any loss of consciousness	Coma, unresponsive, decerebrate
Systolic blood pressure (or central pulse)	>90 mm Hg Good peripheral pulses	50-90 mm Hg Weak carotid/femoral pulse palpable	<50 mm Hg Very weak or no pulses
Skeletal (fractures)	None seen or suspected	Single closed fracture anywhere or suspected	Open or multiple fractures
Open wounds	No visible injury	Minor contusion, abrasion, laceration <7 cm not through fascia, burns <10% and not involving hands, face, feet, or genitalia	Major/penetrating tissue loss, any gunshot wound or stab through fascia; burns >10% or involving hands, face, feet, or genitalia

Scoring: 9-12 = Minor trauma; 6-8 = Potentially life threatening; 0-5 = Life threatening; <0 = Usually fatal

FOCUSED HISTORY–TRAUMA PATIENT

Remember to use age-appropriate language when asking questions of the patient.

In addition to the SAMPLE or CIAMPEDS history, consider the questions in the following list when obtaining a focused history for a pediatric trauma patient. This list will require modification based on the patient's age, mechanism of injury, and patient's chief complaint.

Mechanism of Injury

- How did the injury occur? When?
- Circumstances of the incident—Does the explanation for how the trauma occurred fit the injury and the child's abilities?

Fall Injury

- Height of the fall?
- What type of surface did the child land on?

Motor Vehicle Crash

- Site of impact (e.g., lateral, frontal)? Estimated speed? What was struck (e.g., moving or stationary object)? Amount of damage to the vehicle?
- Where was the child located in the vehicle? Was the child restrained? Was the child's safety seat properly secured?
- Was the vehicle equipped with an air bag? If so, did the air bag deploy (open)?
- Ejected from the vehicle? Prolonged extrication required? Scene fatalities?

Pedestrian Injury

- If the child was struck by a car and thrown while walking, roller-skating, or bicycling, was a helmet worn? If so, is it still in place or was it knocked off the head on impact? Is there damage to the helmet?
- How fast was the car traveling?
- Where was the child struck?
- How far was the child thrown?
- What type of surface did the child land on?

Bicycle Injury

- If struck by a motor vehicle, was the vehicle moving or stationary? If moving, estimated speed?
- Was the child wearing a helmet? If so, is it still in place or was it knocked off the head on impact? Is there damage to the helmet?

Burns

- Location of the burn?
- What caused the burn (e.g., fire, scalding, electrical shock, chemicals)?
- How long ago did the injury occur?
- What treatment has been given?

Penetrating Trauma

- Location of the wound(s)?
- Type/caliber/velocity of the weapon?
- Distance from which the child was shot (close range or long range) or stabbed?
- Presence of powder burns surrounding the wounds?
- Number of shots or stab wounds?
- Estimated blood loss at the scene?

Chronology

- Initial Glasgow Coma Score?
- Behavior immediately after the incident (e.g., crying, stunned, seizure, unconscious)?
- Loss of consciousness immediately or shortly after the incident? Duration?
- Any breathing problems following the injury?

BURN CENTER CRITERIA

- Second-degree burns involving over 10% TBSA in adults or 5% TBSA in children
- Chemical burns
- All burns involving hands, face, eyes, ears, feet, perineum, or circumferential burns of torso or extremities
- Any third degree burn in a child
- All inhalation injuries
- Electrical burns, including lightning injury
- All burns complicated by fractures or other trauma
- All burns in high-risk patients including elderly, very young, those with pre-existing diseases such as diabetes, asthma, and epilepsy

Recommended Childhood and Adolescent Immunization Schedule — United States, 2003

Vaccine ▼	Age ►	Birth	1 mo	2 mos	4 mos	6 mos	12 mos	15 mos	18 mos	24 mos	4-6 yrs	11-12 yrs	13-18 yrs
Hepatitis B		HepB #1 *only if mother HBsAg (–)*											
			HepB #2			HepB #3				HepB series			
Diphtheria, Tetanus, Pertussis				DTaP	DTaP	DTaP		DTaP			DTaP	Td	Td
Haemophilus influenzae Type b				Hib	Hib	Hib	Hib						
Inactivated Polio				IPV	IPV	IPV	IPV				IPV		
Measles, Mumps, Rubella							MMR #1				MMR #2	MMR #2	MMR #2
Varicella							Varicella			Varicella	Varicella		
Pneumococcal				PCV	PCV	PCV	PCV	PCV		PCV	PPV		
Hepatitis A										Hepatitis A series			
Influenza						Influenza (yearly)							

range of recommended ages · catch-up vaccination · preadolescent assessment

Vaccines below this line are for selected populations

Any dose not given at recommended time should be given at any subsequent visit. ■ Indicates catch-up vaccine age groups. Consult www.cdc.gov and the manufacturer's package for full details.

146

Bacterial Meningitis: Presentation By Age

ASSESSMENT FINDINGS	<2-3 MONTHS	2-3 MONTHS TO 2 YEARS	>2 YEARS
Apnea/cyanosis	Common	Rare	Rare
Fever	Common	Common	Common
Hypothermia	Common	Rare	Rare
Altered mental status	Common	Common	Common
Headache	Rare	Rare	Common
Seizures	Early finding	Early finding	Late finding
Ataxia	Rare	Variable	Early finding
Jitteriness	Common	Common	Rare
Vomiting	Common	Common	Variable
Stiff neck	Rare	Late finding	Common
Bulging fontanelle	Common	Common	Closed

Adapted from Barkin RM, Rosen P: Neurologic disorders in emergency pediatrics: A guide to ambulatory care, ed 5, St. Louis, 1999, Mosby.

Possible Causes of Altered Mental Status (AEIOUTIPPS)

A	Alcohol, Abuse
E	Epilepsy, Electrolyte disorders, Encephalopathy, Endocrine
I	Insulin, Intussusception, Intoxication
O	Overdose (opiates, lead, sedatives, aspirin, carbon monoxide)
U	Uremia (kidney failure) and other metabolic causes, Underdosage
T	Trauma, Temperature, Tumor
I	Infection (encephalitis, meningitis, Reye's syndrome, sepsis)
P	Psychological ("fake," "hysterical," or pseudoseizures)
P	Poisoning
S	Shock, Sickle cell disease, Subarachnoid hemorrhage, Space-occupying lesion, Shunt-related problems

HYPOGLYCEMIA

History: Rapid onset, took too much insulin, less food intake than usual, increased exercise

Hunger	Headache
Fatigue	Staring
Irritability	Nausea
Dizziness	Inability to concentrate
Weakness	Diaphoresis
Tachycardia	Incoordination
Agitation	Blurred vision
Tremors	Seizures

HYPERGLYCEMIA

History: Gradual onset (hours to days);
excessive food intake containing sugar,
insufficient insulin dosage

- Altered mental status (varies from
  drowsiness to coma)
- Rapid, deep breathing (Kussmaul respirations)
- Loss of appetite
- Dry skin
- Nausea and/or vomiting
- Normal or slightly decreased blood pressure
- Sweet or fruity (acetone) breath odor
- Thirst
- Abdominal pain
- Tachycardia
- Weakness

Assessment and Management of Pediatric Diabetic Emergencies

ASSESSMENT	HYPOGLYCEMIA	HYPERGLYCEMIA
First impression	• Normal or decreased responsiveness • Pale, diaphoretic	• Normal or decreased responsiveness • Face flushed
Breathing	• Normal to increased rate	• Initial respirations deep, rapid • Late: Kussmaul respirations
Circulation	• Tachycardia • Normal or delayed capillary refill • Normal or cool, pale, clammy skin	• Normal heart rate or tachycardia • Skin dry, warm, flushed
Focused history	• Rapid onset (minutes to hours) • Took too much insulin • Ate less food than usual • Increased exercise • Headache, dizziness, seizures	• Gradual onset (hours to days) • Took too little insulin • Ate excessive food containing sugar • Polyuria, polydipsia, polyphagia
Focused physical examination	• Normal breath odor • Tremors, staring, inability to concentrate, incoordination, irritability	• Possible fruity breath odor • Abdominal pain • Signs of dehydration • Nausea and/or vomiting
Initial management	• ABCs, O_2, IV, dextrose IV or glucagon IM	• ABCs, O_2, IV, fluid challenge for signs of dehydration or shock

RESTRAINING A CHILD*

A Assistance in applying restraints.
   At least four healthcare or law enforcement personnel are needed (at least one for each extremity).

B Body substance isolation precautions. Be careful to avoid contact with bodily fluids.

C Communicate with the patient and family. Constantly monitor the patient.

D Document the reason for restraints, type of restraint used, time placed, status of the patient's airway, breathing, and circulation before and after restraints were applied, reassessments of the patient, and the time removed.

*Adapted from Prendergast HM, Anderson TR: Psychiatric emergencies. In Strange GR, Ahrens WR, Lelyeld S, Schafermeyer RW, editors: Pediatric emergency medicine: a comprehensive study guide, ed 2, American College of Emergency Physicians, New York, 2002, McGraw-Hill.

When applying physical restraints, do not inflict unnecessary pain or use unreasonable force. Never leave a restrained patient unattended. This caution applies to the use of both physical and chemical restraints.

Behavioral Signs of Attention-Deficit/Hyperactivity Disorder

PRESCHOOL (3-5 yrs)	SCHOOL-AGE (6-12 yrs)	ADOLESCENT (13-18 yrs)	ADULT (>18 yrs)
Always on the go	Easily distracted, hard to stay on task	Restless, rather than hyperactive	Multiple jobs, relationships
Aggressive (hits or pushes others)	Homework poorly organized, incomplete, and contains careless errors	School work disorganized and incomplete	Misjudges time available, frequently late
Dangerously daring	Impatient, blurts out answers, fails to wait turn in games	Procrastination on most tasks	Mood lability and flash anger outbursts
Noisy, interrupts	Often out of seat	Engages in risky behavior (speeding, drug experimentation)	Many projects started but few completed
Excessive temper tantrums	Perceived as immature	Poor peer relationships	
Insatiable curiosity		Poor self-esteem	
Low levels of compliance		Difficulty with authority figures	

Adapted from: Dodson WW. Attention Deficit-Hyperactivity Disorder in Jacobson JL: Psychiatric Secrets, 2nd ed., Philadelphia, 2001, Hanley and Belfus.

Signs/Symptoms and Management of Hypothermia

ASSESSMENT	MILD Core temp 93.2° to 96.8° F (34° to 36° C)	MODERATE Core temp 86° to 93° F (30° to 34° C)	SEVERE Core temp <86° F (30° C)
Airway	Patent	Patent	Compromised
Breathing	Normal	Decreased respiratory rate	Slow, shallow, or absent respirations
Circulation	Normal heart rate Normal BP Pale, dry or wet skin	Normal heart rate, bradycardia, atrial fibrillation Normal BP or hypotension Pale, cyanotic, or mottled skin	Osborne waves on ECG Cyanotic or mottled skin Body appears lifeless Spontaneous VF
Mental status	AVPU=A Slurred speech	AVPU=V Decreased responsiveness	AVPU=P or U Extreme disorientation
Other S/S	Shivering Uncoordinated movement	Stiffening muscles Shivering ceases below 86 to 89.6° F	Loss of deep tendon reflexes Stiff, rigid muscles
Initial management	Remove to warm environment Apply warm dry clothing, and blankets Apply radiant heat, warm air, or heat packs	Remove to warm environment Apply warm, dry clothing, and blankets Apply radiant heat, warm air, or heat packs to thorax only	Warm, humidified O₂ Warm IV fluids Continue rewarming until core temperature >95° F (35°C), or return of spontaneous circulation, or resuscitation efforts cease

Signs/Symptoms of Heat-Related Illnesses

ASSESSMENT	HEAT CRAMPS Core temp normal or slightly elevated	HEAT EXHAUSTION Core temp slightly elevated 100.4° F (38° C) to 104° F (40° C)	HEAT STROKE Core temp >104° F (40° C)
Airway	Patent	Patent possible compromise	Compromised
Breathing	Normal	Normal	Varies
Circulation	Normal heart rate or tachycardia Diaphoretic	Tachycardia Diaphoretic Hypotension	Hot, dry, flushed skin pale as condition worsens Weak peripheral pulses with signs of shock
Mental status	AVPU=A	AVPU=V	AVPU=P or U
Other S/S	Painful cramping of abdomen or any extremity	Decreased urine output Headache, body aches Thirst	Muscle stiffness and cramps Seizures Coma

Management of Heat-Related Illnesses

HEAT CRAMPS	HEAT EXHAUSTION	HEAT STROKE
• Remove from hot environment • Rest • Give diluted oral electrolyte solution	• Remove from hot environment • Remove clothing • Ensure patent airway O_2, assist ventilations as needed • If alert, rehydrate with oral fluids • If necessary establish IV/IO access and give an IV fluid bolus 20 mL/kg normal saline or Ringer's lactate • Monitor blood glucose levels; treat hypoglycemia	• Remove from hot environment, remove clothing, cover child in sheets soaked in saline or cold water • Apply cold packs to head, neck, axillae, groin • Ensure patent airway O_2, assist ventilations as needed • Monitor body temperature, discontinue active cooling when child's temperature reaches about 102°F (39°C) • Cardiac monitor • Establish IV/IO access • IV fluid bolus 20 mL/kg normal saline or Ringer's lactate

Near-Drowning: Factors Affecting Patient Outcome

- Duration of the submersion
- Duration and severity of hypoxia
- Water temperature
- Duration and degree of hypothermia
- Diving reflex
- Age of the victim
- Water contamination
- Duration of cardiac arrest
- Promptness of initial treatment
- Response to initial treatment
- Associated injuries (particularly head and cervical spine trauma)

Classification for Submersion Events[13]		
CLINICAL FINDINGS	SEVERITY	MORTALITY (%)
Normal lung auscultation with coughing	1	0
Abnormal lung auscultation with crackles in some lung fields	2	0.6
Abnormal lung auscultation with crackles in all lung fields (acute pulmonary edema) without arterial hypotension	3	5.2
Abnormal lung auscultation with crackles in all lung fields (acute pulmonary edema) with arterial hypotension	4	19.4
Isolated respiratory arrest	5	44
Cardiopulmonary arrest	6	93

Focused History

The history provides critical information in the assessment of the patient with a suspected toxic exposure. In addition to the SAMPLE or CIAMPEDS history, consider the following questions when obtaining a focused history for a patient with a toxic exposure. This list will require modification on the basis of the patient's age and chief complaint.

Critical questions to ask in a toxic exposure situation include what, when, where, why, and how.

- What is the poison?
  - ▶ Determine the exact name of the product, if possible.
  - ▶ Obtain histories from different family members to help confirm the type and dose of exposure.
  - ▶ Are there pill bottles, commercial products, or plants to support the history?
- How was it taken (i.e., ingested, inhaled, absorbed, or injected)?
- When was it taken?
- Where was the child found? How long was the child alone? Any witnesses? Any other children around?
- How much was taken?
  - ▶ Number of pills, amount of liquid
  - ▶ How many/how much available before ingestion?
  - ▶ How many/how much now in the container?
  - ▶ Where is the substance stored?

- What is the child's age? Weight?
- Has the child vomited? How many times?
- What home remedies have been attempted? (Ask specifically about herbal or folk remedies.)
- Has a Poison Control Center been contacted? If so, what instructions were received? What treatment has already been given?
- Has the child been depressed or experienced recent emotional stress?
  - ▶ Divorce, death in the family
  - ▶ Possible suicide attempt in older school-age child or adolescent

▮ TOXINS THAT CAUSE SEIZURES ▮

Amphetamines

Camphor

Isoniazid

Lidocaine

Phenothiazines

Theophylline

Amphetamines

Camphor

Isoniazid

Lidocaine

Phenothiazines

Theophylline

Toxins & Vital Sign Changes

VITAL SIGN	INCREASED	DECREASED
Temperature	Amphetamines anticholinergics, antihistamines, antipsychotic agents, cocaine, monoamine oxidase inhibitors, nicotine, phenothiazines, salicylates, sympathomimetics, theophylline, tricyclic antidepressants, serotonin reuptake inhibitors	Barbiturates, carbon monoxide, clonidine, ethanol, insulin, opiates, oral hypoglycemic agents, phenothiazines, sedative/hypnotics
Pulse	Amphetamines anticholinergics, antihistamines, cocaine, phencyclidine, sympathomimetics, theophylline	Alcohol, beta-blockers, calcium channel blockers, carbamates, clonidine, digoxin, opiates, organophosphates
Respirations	Amphetamines barbiturates (early), caffeine, cocaine, ethylene glycol, methanol, salicylates	Alcohols and ethanol, barbiturates (late), clonidine, opiates, sedative/hypnotics
Blood pressure	Amphetamines anticholinergics, antihistamines, caffeine, clonidine, cocaine, marijuana, phencyclidine, sympathomimetics, theophylline	Antihypertensives, barbiturates, beta-blockers, calcium channel blockers, clonidine, cyanide, opiates, phenothiazines, sedative/hypnotics, tricyclic antidepressants (late)

Clinical Presentations of Specific Toxidromes

PRESENTATION, AGENTS INVOLVED, AND ANTIDOTES

TOXIDROME	Signs/symptoms	Typical agents	Primary antidote
Anticholinergic	Agitation or reduced responsiveness, tachypnea, tachycardia, slightly elevated temperature, blurred vision, dilated pupils, urinary retention, decreased bowel sounds; dry, flushed skin	Atropine, diphenhydramine, scopolamine	Physostigmine
Cholinergic	Altered mental status, tachypnea, bronchospasm, bradycardia or tachycardia, salivation, constricted pupils, polyuria, defecation, emesis, fever, lacrimation, seizures, diaphoresis	Organophosphate insecticides (malathion), carbamate insecticides (carbaryl), some mushrooms, nerve agents	Atropine
Opioid	Altered mental status, bradypnea or apnea, bradycardia, hypotension, pinpoint pupils, hypothermia	Codeine, fentanyl, heroin, meperidine, methadone, oxycodone, dextromethorphan, propoxyphene	Naloxone

Sedative/Hypnotic	Slurred speech, confusion, hypotension, tachycardia, pupil dilation or constriction, dry mouth, respiratory depression, decreased temperature, delirium, hallucinations, coma, paresthesias, blurred vision, ataxia, nystagmus	Ethanol, anticonvulsants, barbiturates, benzodiazepines	Benzodiazepines: flumazenil
Sympathomimetic	Agitation tachypnea, tachycardia, hypertension. excessive speech and motor activity, tremor, dilated pupils, disorientation, insomnia, psychosis, fever, seizures, diaphoresis	Albuterol, amphetamines (e.g., "ecstasy"), caffeine, cocaine, epinephrine, ephedrine, methamphetamine, phencyclidine, pseudoephedrine	Benzodiazepines

Toxicology Memory Aids

Anticholinergic Syndrome (antihistamines, tricyclic antidepressants)	Mad as a hatter - confused delirium Red as a beet - flushed skin Dry as a bone - dry mouth Hot as Hades - hyperthermia Blind as a bat - dilated pupils
Cholinergic Syndrome (SLUDGE or DUMBELS)	**S**alivation, **L**acrimation, **U**rination, **D**efecation, **G**astrointestinal distress, **E**mesis **D**iarrhea, **U**rination, **M**iosis (pinpoint pupils), **B**ronchospasm/ Bronchorrhea/ **B**radycardia, **E**mesis, **L**acrimation, **S**alivation

Odors and Toxins

ODOR	TOXIN
Acetone	Acetone, isopropyl alcohol, salicylates
Alcohol	Ethanol, isopropyl alcohol
Bitter almonds	Cyanide
Carrots	Water hemlock
Fishy	Zinc or aluminum phosphide
Fruity	Isopropyl alcohol, chlorinated hydrocarbons (e.g., chloroform)
Garlic	Arsenic, organophosphates, DMSO, phosphorus, thallium
Glue	Toluene
Mothballs	Camphor
Pears	Chloral hydrate, paraldehyde
Rotten eggs	Sulfur dioxide, hydrogen sulfide
Shoe polish	Nitrobenzene
Vinyl	Ethchlorvynol
Wintergreen	Methyl salicylates

Toxins and Antidotes

TOXIN	ANTIDOTE
Acetaminophen	N-Acetylcysteine (NAC, Mucomyst)
Arsenic, mercury, other metals	BAL in oil (dimercaprol)
Benzodiazepines	Flumazenil (Romazicon)
Beta-blockers	Glucagon
Calcium channel blockers	Calcium chloride, calcium gluconate, glucagon
Carbon monoxide	Oxygen, hyperbaric oxygen
Coumadin	Vitamin K
Cyanide thiosulfate	Amyl nitrite, sodium nitrite, sodium
Digitalis glycosides	Digoxin-specific Fab antibodies (Digibind)
Iron	Deferoxamine (Desferal)
Isoniazid	Pyridoxine (vitamin B_6)
Lead	EDTA, BAL, DMSA
Methanol, ethylene glycol	Ethanol (ethyl alcohol), Fomepizole (4-MP)
Methemoglobinemia	Methylene blue
Opiates	Naloxone (Narcan)
Organophosphate/ carbamate pesticides	Atropine, pralidoxime (2-PAM, Protopam)
Tricyclic antidepressants	Sodium bicarbonate

Selected Poisonous Plants

PLANT NAME	TOXIN
Black henbane	Anticholinergic
Castor bean	Mimics septic shock; ricin (obtained from castor beans) is used in chemical warfare
Deadly nightshade	Gastric irritation, fever, diarrhea
Dieffenbachia (dumb cane, mother-in-laws tongue, dumb plant, tuft root)	Mucous membranes of mouth typically affected with severe pain, swelling, and sensation of biting into glass
Foxglove	Cardiovascular toxin
Holly	Has 5 toxins; nausea, vomiting, abdominal cramping, diarrhea
Jimsonweed	Anticholinergic; 50 to 100 seeds = 3 to 6 mg atropine
Lily of the valley	Cardiovascular toxin
Mandrake	Anticholinergic; ripe fruit nontoxic
Oleander	Cardiovascular toxin
Philodendron	More than 200 varieties of this popular houseplant; mild oral mucosal irritation, GI upset
Poison hemlock	Nicotine-like toxin; professed to be used in execution of Socrates
Pokeweed (unripe berries)	Berries edible when cooked correctly: "poke salad"; nausea, GI cramps, diaphoresis, emesis, diarrhea
Rhododendron	Includes over 1000 species of azaleas and rhododendrons, including mountain laurel, dwarf laurel, rose bay, western Labrador tea, and Japanese pieris; cardiovascular toxin; bradycardia, hypotension, nausea, vomiting, abdominal pain
Rhubarb	Renal toxin; stalks are edible
Tobacco plants	Nicotine-like toxin
Water hemlock	Neurotoxin; seizures = severe toxicity and a common cause of death
Yellow oleander	Cardiovascular toxin
Yew	Cardiovascular toxin; dizziness, dry mouth, nausea, emesis, rash, cyanosis, coma, bradycardia, dysrhythmias
Pitted fruits (e.g., apricot seeds, bitter almonds, peach kernels) —chewed pits	Contain a plant compound that contains sugar and produces cyanide; cyanosis, difficulty breathing, vomiting, weakness, coma, seizures, cardiovascular collapse

RISK FOR MALTREATMENT

CHILD RISK FACTORS

- Premature birth or neonatal separation
- Congenital defect
- Developmental disability
- Physical disability
- Chronic illness
- Multiple birth

CAREGIVER RISK FACTORS

- Often abused as a child
- Young maternal age
- History of mental illness or criminal activity
- Financial stress, unemployment
- Physical illness of parent or child
- Marital or relationship stress
- Low self-esteem, depression
- Substance abuse

■■■ CHARACTERISTICS OF ABUSERS ■■■

- Shows little concern for the child's injury, treatment, or prognosis
- Denies the existence of (or blames the child for) the child's problems in school or at home
- Seldom touches or looks at the child
- Has little perception of how a child could feel, physically or emotionally
- Asks teachers or other caregivers to use harsh physical discipline if the child misbehaves
- Sees the child as entirely bad, worthless, or burdensome
- Demands a level of physical or academic performance the child cannot achieve
- Looks primarily to the child for care, attention, and satisfaction of emotional needs

■■■ CHARACTERISTICS OF ABUSE ■■■

- Accidental versus intentional injury
  - ▶ Children are often injured; however, not all children with injuries are abused.
  - ▶ Child abuse is unlikely if the child's story is volunteered without hesitation and matches that of the caregiver.
  - ▶ Distinguishing between an intentional injury and an accident is a challenge.
- Signs that may signal the presence of child abuse or neglect
  - ▶ Cries hopelessly during treatment or cries very little in general
  - ▶ Shows sudden changes in behavior or school performance
  - ▶ May constantly seek favors, food, or things

- ▶ Has not received help for physical or medical problems brought to the parents' attention
- ▶ Does not look at caregiver for reassurance
- ▶ Has learning problems (or difficulty in concentrating) that cannot be attributed to specific physical or psychological causes
- ▶ Is always watchful, as though preparing for something bad to happen
- ▶ Lacks adult supervision
- ▶ Is overly compliant, passive, or withdrawn
- ▶ Comes to school or other activities early, stays late, and does not want to go home

INDICATORS OF NEGLECT

- Missed medical appointments
- Failure or delay in seeking medical care for illness or injuries
- Failure or delay in seeking dental care
- Poor growth
- Poor hygiene
- Failure to thrive
- Untreated medical conditions
- Lack of adult supervision
- Inappropriate or inadequate clothing
- Unsafe living environment
- Malnourished appearing child
- Lack of necessary immunizations
- Failure to provide required medication (e.g., asthmatic with no medication)

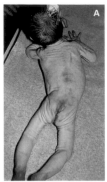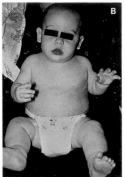

Failure to thrive as a result of neglect. **A**, This 4½-month-old infant was brought to an emergency department because of congestion. She was found to be below her birth weight and suffering from severe developmental delay. Note the marked loss of subcutaneous tissue manifested by the wrinkled skin folds over her buttocks, shoulders, and upper arms. **B**, 3½ months after removal from the home, she was well nourished and had caught up developmentally.

PHYSICAL ABUSE

PHYSICAL INDICATORS OF ABUSE

- Over 90% of child abuse cases involve injuries to skin
- Injuries can be anywhere: important factor is distribution
- Bruises and welts
  - ▸ Accidental bruises tend to be small and nonspecific in configuration, usually at protuberant areas, such as the chin, cheek bone, and forehead. Bruises on the cheeks, abdomen, back, buttocks, and inner thigh should raise suspicion.
  - ▸ Pattern suggestive of object used (e.g., hand, wire hanger, rope, belt buckle, human bite marks, pinch marks)

- ► Multiple bruises in various stages of healing
  - ○ In general, a fresh injury is red to blue
  - ○ 1-3 days, deep black or purple
  - ○ 3-6 days, green changing to brown
  - ○ 6-15 days, green to tan to yellow to faded, then disappears
- ► Other explanations for bruises
  - ○ Mongolian spots—benign and not associated with any conditions or illnesses
  - ○ Ehlers-Danlos syndrome (EDS)—fragility of skin is common, with frequent bruises and lacerations
  - ○ Coagulation disorders such as hemophilia, von Willebrand's disease, thrombocytopenic purpura, or leukemia

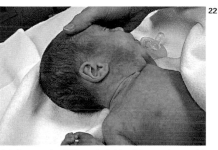

22

Facial slap marks. Diffuse facial bruising and petechiae seen over the side of the face and head of this 3-week-old infant were the result of slaps by his father, a paranoid schizophronic who had stopped taking his medication. He acknowledged slapping his son to make him cry, after which he would give him his bottle. The "purpose" was to teach him to cry when hungry.

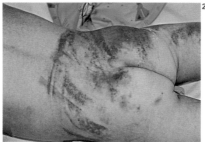

The severe contusions on the buttocks and lower back of this child were inflicted by hand, hairbrush, and belt.

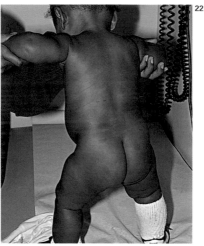

Mongolian spots. This toddler, referred from a daycare center because of "multiple bruises," actually had an unusual number of Mongolian spots.

- Human bite marks
  - Strongly suggest abuse; easily over-looked
  - Location on infants tends to be on the genitals and buttocks
    - Usually inflicted as punishment
  - Older children tend to have bite marks that are associated with assault or sexual abuse
    - There are generally more than one, occur at random, appearance is well-defined, and they may be associated with a sucking mark
- Burns
  - Inflicted burns
    - Most common inflicted burn injury is that caused by immersion in scalding water
    - "Glove-like" or "stocking-like" burns with no associated splash marks
    - Usually present on the buttocks, perineum, genitalia, or extremities
    - Often associated with toilet training
    - Average age of the victim is approximately 2 years

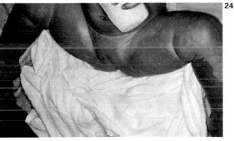

24

Inflicted scald. This toddler was dipped in scalding water while being held under the arms and knees, as an object lesson following a toileting accident.

- Circular burns from a cigarette or cigar
- Rope burns on wrists from being bound
- Burns in the shape of a household utensil or appliance (e.g., heated fork, spoon, iron)

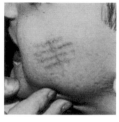

22

These facial burns are the result of being branded with the grille of a hair dryer. The boy had been acting out while he was supposed to be getting ready for school and his mother was drying her hair.

► Other explanations for burns
- Impetigo (a contagious bacterial skin infection) may resemble a burn
- Chickenpox may resemble cigarette burns
- Burns caused by hot areas of a child safety seat may be mistaken for an abusive injury

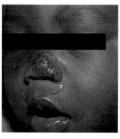

22

Impetigo. This infant was initially suspected of having a cigar burn, but close inspection revealed a new peripheral bullous rim. This and the presence of another early impetiginous lesion on the cheek enabled the correct diagnosis to be made.

- Fractures
  - Suspicious fractures
    - Fractures that are "accidentally" discovered during assessment of the child
    - Skeletal injury out of proportion with the history provided
    - Multiple fractures that are symmetrical or in different stages of healing
    - Skeletal trauma accompanied by injuries (e.g., burns) to other parts of the body
- Hair loss
  - Pulling of the child's hair and then dragging the child may cause traumatic alopecia (baldness)
  - Blood beneath or at the surface of the scalp can help differentiate abusive versus nonabusive traumatic hair loss
- Head, face, and oral injuries
  - Unintentional injuries to the face or head usually involve the front of the body
  - Injuries to the sides of the face, ears, cheeks, and temple area are highly suspicious of abuse
  - Infants may sustain injuries during feeding by having a spoon or other object forced into the mouth
  - A torn frenulum may indicate forcing a nipple from a bottle or pacifier into the child's mouth
  - Head injury occurs as a result of:
    - Vigorous shaking of an infant (shaken baby syndrome)
    - Pressure on the carotid arteries of the neck during shaking, resulting in decreased oxygenation of the brain and swelling

- A direct blow to the head—the infant is both shaken and struck on the head (shaken impact syndrome)
- Rib fractures and grip marks on the extremities may be present from violent shaking
- Child may experience apnea or seizures, and/or may be slow to respond
- Abdominal injuries
  - Child may be punched or kicked in the abdomen.
  - Because the child's abdominal wall is elastic and absorbs much of the force, only mild bruising may be seen or there may be no external sign of injury.
  - Child may experience abdominal tenderness, vomiting, and/or signs of shock.

REPORTING REQUIREMENTS

Each state and U.S. territory designates individuals, typically by professional group, who are mandated by law to report child maltreatment. Any person, however, may report incidents of abuse or neglect.

PERSONS TYPICALLY MANDATED TO REPORT

- Persons typically designated as mandatory reporters have frequent contact with children. Such individuals include:
  - Healthcare workers
  - School personnel
  - Child care providers
  - Social workers
  - Law enforcement officers
  - Mental health professionals

- Some states also mandate animal control officers, veterinarians, commercial film or photograph processors, substance abuse counselors, and firefighters to report abuse or neglect. Four states (Alaska, Arkansas, Connecticut, and South Dakota) include domestic violence workers on the list of mandated reporters. Approximately 18 states require all citizens to report suspected abuse or neglect regardless of profession.

DOCUMENTATION

Document the caregiver's comments exactly as stated and enclose in quotation marks.

Documentation should include:

- Description of the scene
  - General appearance of the home and other children
  - Appearance of the room where the injury occurred
  - Any unusual, unsafe, or unsanitary conditions
  - Behavior of those present at the scene
- History of the injury or illness
  - Document the when, where, and how regarding the injury
  - Document who was present
  - Indicate any discrepancies in statements in the record
    - Statements made by the caregivers should be documented exactly as stated and noted in quotation marks
- Findings from the physical examination
  - Objectively document physical examination findings including the type, number, size, and location of injuries
  - Document any pattern of injury, if observed

ABUSE ASSESSMENT

Physical Abuse

PHYSICAL FINDINGS	SUGGESTIVE BEHAVIORS
• Bruises and welts, wounds at different stages of healing • Burns, especially on feet, palms of hands, back and buttocks; absence of splash mark • Fractures and dislocations—skull, nose, facial; fracture with spiral fracture or dislocation • Any injury not consistent with history • Lacerations and abrasions on back of arms, torso, face, or external genitalia • Bites or pulling out of hair • Unexplained poisonings or chemical exposures	• Wariness of physical contact with adults • Apparent fear of parents or of going home • Inappropriate reaction to injury such as failure to cry from pain • Lack of reactions to frightening events • Superficial relationships • Apprehension when hearing other children cry • Withdrawal or acting out behavior

Physical Neglect

PHYSICAL FINDINGS	SUGGESTIVE BEHAVIORS
• Failure to thrive • Malnutrition, lack of subcutaneous fat • Poor personal hygiene • Unclean and/or inappropriate dress • Evidence of poor health care • Frequent illnesses or injury	• Dull and inactive, passive or sleepy • Self-stimulatory behaviors, finger sucking, rocking • Begging/stealing food • Absenteeism from school • Drug/alcohol addiction • Vandalism/shoplifting

Tables on p. 176-177 from *Mosby's Nursing PDQ*:
St. Louis, 2004, Mosby.

Emotional Abuse/Neglect

PHYSICAL FINDINGS	SUGGESTIVE BEHAVIORS
• Failure to thrive • Feeding disorders • Enuresis • Sleep disorders	• Self-stimulatory behaviors, finger sucking, rocking, biting • Withdrawal • Unusual fearfulness • Antisocial behavior • Lag in emotional or intellectual development • Suicide attempt

Sexual Abuse

PHYSICAL FINDINGS	SUGGESTIVE BEHAVIORS
• Bruises, bleeding, lacerations or irritation to external genitalia, anus, mouth, or throat • Torn, stained, bloody underclothing • Pain on urination or pain, swelling, and itching of genital area • Penile discharge • Sexually transmitted infection • Difficulty walking or sitting • Unusual odor in genital area • Recurrent urinary tract infection • Evidence of semen • Pregnancy in young adolescent	• Sudden emergence of sexually related problems, sexual play, excessive masturbation, seductive behavior • Withdrawn behavior, excessive daydreaming • Preoccupation with fantasies • Poor relationship with peers • Sudden changes—anxiety, weight loss/gain, clinging behavior • Regressive behaviors—bed-wetting, thumb-sucking • Running away from home • Profound personality change • Suicide attempts or ideation

PREVENTING SUDDEN INFANT DEATH SYNDROME (SIDS)

- Place an infant supine for sleep.
- "Back to sleep" or "face up to wake up."
- Side sleeping is not recommended.
- Place an infant on a firm surface for sleep. Avoid soft or padded sleep surfaces (e.g., pillows, sheepskins, sofas, soft mattresses, waterbeds, beanbag cushions, quilts, comforters).
- Avoid soft materials (e.g., pillows, comforters, quilts, sheepskins, and stuffed toys) over, under, or near the infant's sleep environment If used, blankets should be tucked in around the crib mattress.
- Do not overbundle or dress the infant too warmly.
- Avoid exposure to cigarette smoke.
- Other than parents, no one should share a bed with an infant. Parents who smoke, drink, or use drugs should not share a bed with their infant because the substances may impair their reflexes.

Risk Factors for SIDS[14]	
MATERNAL	**INFANT**
• Young age	• Male gender
• Multiparity	• Low birth weight
• Smoking during pregnancy	• Low birth length
• Maternal drug abuse	• Premature birth
• Previous fetal deaths	• Blood type B
• Anemia during pregnancy	• Low Apgar scores
• Low social class	• Low hematocrit at 48 hours
• Low family income	• Prone sleeping position
• Short interpregnancy interval	• Overheating
• Unmarried mother	• Not breastfed
• Late attendance of antenatal clinic	• Previous cyanotic episode
• Postnatal depression	• Previous SIDS in family
• Attendance to psychiatrist	

SIDS History and Documentation

QUESTIONS	OBSERVATIONS AT THE SCENE
• What is the baby's name? • What happened? • What is baby's* age? • What does baby weigh? • What time was baby put to bed? • When did baby fall asleep? • Who last saw baby alive? • Who found baby? What did that person do? • What position was baby in when he/she was found? • Was CPR attempted? • Did baby share a bed with anyone else? • What was the general health of baby? • Had baby been ill recently? • Was baby taking any medications?	• Position and location of the infant on arrival • General appearance of the home and other children, appearance of the room where the death occurred, condition and characteristics of the crib or sleep area • Bedding (e.g., pillows, sheets, blankets, etc.), any objects in the crib (e.g., toys or bottles), or any unusual or dangerous items that could cause choking or suffocation • Medications • Electrical and mechanical devices in use in the room including vaporizers, space heaters, fans, and infant electronic monitors (e.g., apnea monitor or heart rate monitor) • Behavior of those present at the scene

*Substitute the infant's name for "baby."

Coping With the Death of an Infant or Child

CAREGIVER REACTION	INTERVENTION/RESPONSE
Shock, denial ("This can't be happening.")	
• Suddenness of the death left no time for preparation or goodbyes • Difficult to comprehend the death of an infant who did not appear to be sick • Inability or refusal to believe the reality of the event • Numbness, repression of emotional response	• Allow caregivers to express their grief • Refer to infant by name and encourage caregivers to talk about the baby • Provide an opportunity for the caregivers to see and hold infant's body • Do not say, "Time heals . . ."
Guilt ("If only I had . . ." "If only I had checked on the baby sooner." "If only I had taken the baby to the doctor with that slight cold.")	
• Caregivers often feel guilty about not being with the infant at the time of the incident to prevent it from happening or feel that the infant's death was their fault	• Provide reassurance that caregiver did not cause the infant's death • Encourage caregivers to ask questions • Keep answers to questions as brief as possible • Do not say, "This happened because . . ."
Anger ("Why my baby?")	
• Caregiver's anger is related to his or her inability to control or change the situation • Anger is displaced and projected to anything and everything	• Do not take anger or insults personally • Be tolerant and empathetic • Do not become defensive • Use good listening and communication skills • Do not say, "I know how you feel."
Helplessness, frustration ("What am I going to do?" "Why is this happening to me?")	
• Surfacing of painful feelings • Caregiver feels alone, disconnected, and alienated	• Ensure availability of a family friend, relative, or religious representative to provide further support • Encourage participation in local SIDS program support services • Do not say, "You can still have other children."

▆ DISORDERS AND DISABILITIES ▆

Examples of disorders and diseases of children with special healthcare needs:

- Deformities present at birth or acquired, such as club feet, dislocated hip, cleft palate, malunited fractures, scoliosis, spina bifida, and congenital GU and GI anomalies
- Heart conditions resulting from congenital deformities or from rheumatic fever
- Cerebral palsy
- Cystic fibrosis
- Sickle cell anemia
- Hemophilia
- Neurofibromatosis
- Hydrocephalus
- Rheumatoid arthritis
- Many muscle and nerve disorders
- Some conditions of epilepsy
- Cancer
- Premature infant
- Diabetes

COGNITIVE DISABILITIES

- Cognitive disabilities affect awareness, memory, and ability to learn, process information, communicate, and make decisions.

Special Needs

- ▶ A child may have associated deficits such as motor impairment, behavioral/emotional disorder, medical complications, or seizure disorder.
- The physical examination of a child with a cognitive disability is no different from that of other children, but the child's ability to communicate and understand will be affected. The degree of impairment will vary depending on the child's age, the child's illness or injury, and the severity of the disability.

PHYSICAL DISABILITIES

- A physical disability involves some type of mobility limitation.
- Conditions such as cerebral palsy, spina bifida, and muscular dystrophy often involve mobility limitations.
- The child may use a corrective splint, wheelchair, braces, crutches, or other device to enhance mobility.

A child with special healthcare needs who has any of the following conditions should be considered unstable or critical:

- Partial or total airway obstruction in children with tracheostomies
- Respiratory difficulties in ventilator-dependent children
- Bradycardia, irregular pulses, or signs of compensated shock in children with pacemakers
- Fever, nausea, vomiting, headache, or a change in mental status in children with CSF shunts
- Signs of worsening illness despite appropriate home therapy in any child with a chronic health problem

Since ventilator-dependent children always require assisted ventilation, critical status applies only if one or more additional signs are present.

Causes of CSF Shunt Malfunction

D Displacement (catheter migration), disconnection of shunt components, drainage —overdrainage or inadequate drainage

O Obstructed or fractured catheter, kinking of distal catheter

P Perforated abdominal viscus, peritonitis, pseudocyst

E Erosion of the equipment through the skin

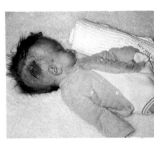

External shunt infection in a premature infant with poor nutritional status.

Complications of Enteral Feeding Tubes

- Wound infection
  Pulmonary aspiration of formula

- Dehydration
  Electrolyte imbalance

- Tube obstruction
  Tube dislodgement

- Peritonitis
  Leakage around the tube

- Bowel obstruction
  Nausea, diarrhea

Routes of drainage for ventriculoperitoneal (VP) and ventriculoatrial (VA) shunts.

VP shunts (left) drain cerebrospinal fluid (CSF) from the cerebral ventricles via catheter tubing implanted superficially over the rib cage. The lower end of the peritoneal catheter lies free in the abdomen.

VA shunts (right) drain CSF to the right atrium via the superior vena cava or the jugular vein.

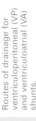

■ TRACHEOSTOMY OBSTRUCTION ■

- Altered mental status with restlessness, agitation
- Increased work of breathing
- Raspy noises from tracheostomy tube during respiration
- Change in sounds during respiration
- Diminished breath sounds
- Nasal flaring, retractions
- Difficulty eating or sucking
- Decreased O_2 saturation
- Marked use of accessory muscles
- Poor peripheral perfusion; mottling
- Tachycardia (bradycardia is a late sign)
- Inadequate chest rise during spontaneous or assisted ventilation
- High peak pressure alarm on ventilator
- Difficulty in ventilating when providing assisted ventilation
- Cyanosis, bradycardia, and unresponsiveness (late findings)

■ TRACHEOSTOMY SUCTIONING ■

- Indication by the patient that suctioning is necessary
- Suspected aspiration of gastric or upper airway secretions
- Visible secretions in the airway; secretions bubbling in the tracheostomy tube
- Wheezes, crackles, or gurgling on inspiration or expiration audible to the patient and/or caregiver with or without auscultation
- More frequent or congested-sounding cough

- Patient's inability to clear secretions by coughing
- Altered mental status, restlessness or irritability
- Unexplained increase in work of breathing, respiratory rate, or heart rate
- Decrease in vital capacity and/or O_2 saturation
- Unilateral or bilateral absent or diminished breath sounds
- Cyanosis

VENTILATOR EMERGENCIES

If a child attached to a ventilator shows signs of respiratory distress, identification and treatment of possible causes is important. The DOPE mnemonic can be used to recall possible reversible causes of acute deterioration in an intubated child.

- **D**isplaced tube (e.g., right mainstem or esophageal intubation) or **D**isconnection of the tube or ventilator circuit—reassess tube position, ventilator connections
- **O**bstructed tube (e.g., blood or secretions are obstructing air flow)—suction
- **P**neumothorax (tension)—needle thoracostomy
- **E**quipment problem/failure (e.g., empty oxygen source, inadvertent change in ventilator settings, low battery)—check equipment and oxygen source

THE NEWLY BORN

Newborn Assessment and Treatment

Apgar Scoring System			
	0	**1**	**2**
Appearance	Blue, pale	Body pink Extremities blue	Completely pink
Pulse	Absent	<100	100
Grimace/reflex irritability	No response	Grimaces, cries	Cough, sneeze, vigorous cry
Activity/ muscle tone	Limp, flaccid	Some flexion of extremities	Active motion
Respiratory effort	Absent	Slow, irregular	Good, crying

Problems that May Disrupt the Normal Transition to Uterine Life	
PROBLEM	**POSSIBLE RESULT**
Newborn does not breathe sufficiently to force fluid from alveoli	Lungs do not fill with air; oxygen is not available to blood circulating through the lungs→ hypoxia, cyanosis
Meconium blocks air from entering alveoli	
Insufficient blood return from placenta before or during birth	Systemic hypotension
Poor cardiac contractility	
Bradycardia due to insufficient delivery of oxygen to heart or brainstem	
Lack of oxygen or failure to distend lungs with air may result in sustained constriction of pulmonary arterioles	Persistent pulmonary hypertension
Insufficient oxygen delivery to brain	Depressed respiratory drive
Insufficient oxygen delivery to brain and muscles	Poor muscle tone

INITIAL STEPS OF RESUSCITATION OF THE NEWLY BORN

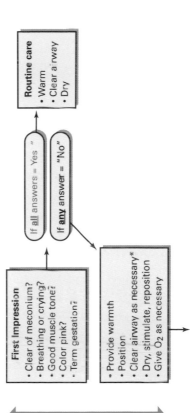

Birth

First Impression
- Clear of meconium?
- Breathing or crying?
- Good muscle tone?
- Color pink?
- Term gestation?

If **all** answers = Yes "

If **any** answer = "No"

Routine care
- Warm
- Clear a rway
- Dry

- Provide warmth
- Position
- Clear airway as necessary*
- Dry, stimulate, reposition
- Give O₂ as necessary

30 seconds

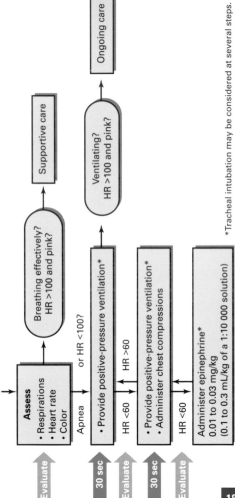

Assess
- Respirations
- Heart rate
- Color

Apnea *or* HR <100?

Breathing effectively? HR >100 and pink? → Supportive care

- Provide positive-pressure ventilation*

Ventilating? HR >100 and pink? → Ongoing care

HR <60

- Provide positive-pressure ventilation*
- Administer chest compressions

HR >60

HR <60

Administer epinephrine* 0.01 to 0.03 mg/kg (0.1 to 0.3 mL/kg of a 1:10 000 solution)

Evaluate — 30 sec — **Evaluate** — 30 sec — **Evaluate**

*Tracheal intubation may be considered at several steps.

189

Laryngoscope Blade and Tracheal Tube Size Based on Age and Weight

WEIGHT (g)	GESTATIONAL AGE (weeks)	LARYNGOSCOPE BLADE SIZE	LARYNGOSCOPE BLADE TYPE	TRACHEAL TUBE SIZE (mm)	DEPTH OF TRACHEAL TUBE INSERTION (cm from upper lip)
<1000	<28	0	Straight	2.5	6.5 to 7.0
1000 to 2000	28 to 34	0	Straight	2.5 to 3.0	7.0 to 8.0
2000 to 3000	34 to 33	0 to 1	Straight	3.0 to 3.5	8.0 to 9.0
>3000	>38	1	Straight	3.5 to 4.0	>9.0

Common Medications

MEDICATION	INDICATIONS	MECHANISM OF ACTION	DOSAGE	NOTES
Glucose	Documented and symptomatic hypoglycemia	Rapidly increases serum glucose concentration reverses CNS effects of hypoglycemia	IV/IO: 200 mg/kg (2 mL/kg of a D10W solution) slow IV push	Hypoglycemia = glucose level less than 40 mg/dl if >2.5 kg, or less than 30 mg/dl if <2.5 kg. Higher concentrations of glucose (e.g., D25W) are hyperosmolar and should be avoided. Repeat glucose measurement should be obtained 10 to 20 minutes after glucose administration.
Sodium bicarbonate	Persistent metabolic acidosis or hyperkalemia (use should be directed by arterial blood gas results or serum chemistries)	Alkalinizing agent	IV: 1 to 2 mEq/kg of a 0.5 mEq/mL solution may be given by slow IV push (over at least 2 minutes) after adequate ventilation and perfusion have been established	Do NOT use during brief resuscitation episodes; hyperosmolarity and CO_2-generating properties may be detrimental to myocardial or cerebral function.

Medications Used in Neonatal Resuscitation

MEDICATION	INDICATIONS	MECHANISM OF ACTION	DOSAGE	NOTES
Epinephrine	Asystole or when the heart rate remains <60 beats/minute after a minimum of 30 seconds of adequate ventilation and chest compressions	Has both alpha and beta-adrenergic stimulating properties. In cardiac arrest, alpha-adrenergic mediated vasoconstriction may be the more important action. Vasoconstriction elevates the perfusion pressure during chest compressions, enhancing delivery of oxygen to the heart and brain. Epinephrine also enhances myocardial contractility, stimulates spontaneous contractions, and increases heart rate.	IV/IO/ET: 0.01 to 0.03 mg/kg (0.1 to 0.3 mL/kg of a 1:10 000 solution), repeated every 3 to 5 minutes as indicated	Available data regarding effects of high-dose epinephrine for resuscitation of newborn infants is inadequate to support routine use of higher doses of epinephrine.

| Naloxone | Reversal of respiratory depression in newly born infant whose mother received narcotics within 4 hours of delivery | Competes with opioid receptor sites in the central nervous system, displacing previously administered narcotic analgesics. | IV/IO/IM/subq : 0.1 mg/kg of a 0.4 mg/mL or 1.0 mg/mL solution | Establish and maintain adequate ventilation before administration. Avoid if mother is suspected of having recently abused narcotics. Administration of naloxone to these newborns may precipitate abrupt withdrawal signs. Repeated doses of naloxone may be necessary to prevent recurrent apnea because duration of action of narcotics may exceed that of naloxone. |

REFERENCES

1. Foltin GL, Tunik MG, Cooper A, Markenson D, Treiber M, Skomorowsky A: *Teaching resource for instructors in prehospital pediatrics for paramedics.* New York, 2002, Center for Pediatric Emergency Medicine.

2. Bower CM: The surgical airway. In Dieckmann RA, Fiser DH, Selbst SM, editors: *Illustrated textbook of pediatric emergency and critical care procedures,* St. Louis, 1997, Mosby.

3. Gerardi MG: Evaluation and management of the multiple trauma patient. In Strange GR, Ahrens WR, Lelyveld S, Schafermeyer RW, editors: *Evaluation and management of the multiple trauma patient in pediatric emergency medicine: A comprehensive study guide,* ed 2, New York, 2002, McGraw-Hill.

4. *CPR pro for the professional rescuer,* 2003, National Instructor's Resource Center, Inc., p. 18.

5. Samson RA, Berg RA, Bingham R; Pediatric Advanced Life Support Task Force, International Liaison Committee on Resuscitation for the American Heart Association; European Resuscitation Council: Use of automated external defibrillators for children: An update — An advisory statement from the Pediatric Advanced Life Support Task Force, International Liaison Committee on Resuscitation. *Pediatrics* 112(1 Pt 1):163-168, 2003.

6. The Use of AEDs for Children. In *CPR pro for the professional rescuer,* 2003, National Instructor's Resource Center, Inc., p. 20.

7. Merskey H, Bogduk N, editors: International Association for the Study of Pain (IASP) Task Force on Taxonomy. *Classification of chronic pain,* ed 2, Seattle, 1994, IASP Press, pp. 209-214.

8. McCaffery M, Pasero CL: When the physician prescribes a placebo, *Am J Nurs* 98(1):52-53, 1998.

9. Wong DL, Hess CS: *Wong and Whaley's clinical manual of pediatric nursing,* ed 5, St. Louis, 2000, Mosby.

10. Woods WA, Mellick LB: Pediatric cervical spine injuries: avoiding potential disaster, *Trauma Reports*, July-August, 2003. http://www.findarticles.com/cf_dls/m0KHW/4_4/105044638/print.jhtml Accessed 12/7/2003.

11. Barkin RM, Rosen P: *Emergency pediatrics: a guide to ambulatory care*, 5e. St. Louis, 1999, Mosby.

12. Bledsoe BE, Clayden DE, Papa FJ: *Prehospital emergency pharmacology*, ed. 4, Upper Saddle River, NJ,1996, Prentice Hall

13. Szpilman D: Near-drowning and drowning classification: A proposal to stratify mortality based on the analysis of 1,831 cases. *Chest* 112(3):660-665, Sep 1997. PMID: 9315798.

14. Poets CF, Southhall DP: Sudden infant death syndrome and apparent life-threatening events. In Taussig LM, Landau LI, editors: *Pediatric respiratory medicine*, St. Louis, 1999, Mosby.

15. Adapted from Tepas JJ III, Mollitt DL, Talbert JL: The pediatric trauma score as a predictor of injury severity in the injured child, *J Pediatr Surg* 22(1):14-8.1987.

16. Behrman RE, Kliegman RM, Jenson HB (ed.) History and Physical Examination in Nelson Textbook of Pediatrics, 16e. Philadelphia, 2000, Saunders.

ILLUSTRATION CREDITS

17. Seidel H, Ball J, Dains J, Benedict GW: *Mosby's guide to physical examination*, ed 5, St Louis, 2003, Mosby.

18. EMSC Slide Set (CD-ROM). 1996. Courtesy of the Emergency Medical Services for Children Program, administered by the U.S. Department of Health and Human Service's Health Resources and Services Administration, Maternal and Child Health Bureau.

19. Aehlert B: *Pediatric advanced life support study guide*, ed 2, St Louis, 2005, Mosby.

20. Dieckmann R, Fiser D, Selbst: *Illustrated textbook of pediatric emergency and critical care procedures*, St. Louis, 1997, Mosby.

21. Hockenberry M: *Wong's essentials of pediatric nursing*, ed 7, St. Louis, 2005, Mosby.
22. Zitelli B, Davis H: *Atlas of pediatric physical diagnosis*, ed 4, St. Louis, 2002, Mosby.
23. Courtesy Dr. Kent Hymel, Falls Church, VA.
24. Courtesy Dr. Thomas Layton.
25. Herlihy B, *The human body in health and illness*, 2e, St. Louis, 2003, Saunders.
26. Cohen J, Powderly W: *Infectious diseases*, 2e, Philadelphia, 2004, Saunders.